REABLEMENT SERVICES IN HEALTH AND SOCIAL CARE

REABLEMENT SERVICES IN HEALTH AND SOCIAL CARE

A GUIDE TO PRACTICE FOR STUDENTS AND SUPPORT WORKERS

VALERIE A. EBRAHIMI

HAZEL M. CHAPMAN

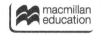 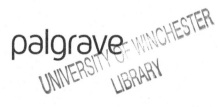

First published 2018 by
PALGRAVE

Palgrave in the UK is an imprint of Macmillan Publishers Limited, registered in England, company number 785998, of 4 Crinan Street, London N1 9XW.

Palgrave® and Macmillan® are registered trademarks in the United States, the United Kingdom, Europe and other countries.

ISBN 978–1–137–37264–2 paperback

This book is printed on paper suitable for recycling and made from fully managed and sustained forest sources. Logging, pulping and manufacturing processes are expected to conform to the environmental regulations of the country of origin.

A catalogue record for this book is available from the British Library.

A catalog record for this book is available from the Library of Congress.

CONTENTS

LIST OF BOXES, FIGURES AND TABLES

Boxes

Figures

Tables

LIST OF ACTIVITIES AND SCENARIOS

Student Activities

List of Reflection Points

Scenarios

Sá einn veit sem reynir
You won't know, until you give it a go…

CONTRIBUTORS

VALERIE A. EBRAHIMI (aka Vala Viðarsdóttir)

Starting out in 1995 as an assistant to inspiring Occupational Therapists (OT) in Reykjavik, Vala moved to Scotland in 1997. It was there, after continuing to work as a carer and gaining more qualifications that she was finally accepted onto an OT degree in 1998, but not until after persuading Averil Stewart, the first UK Professor Emeritus. Vala's initial post was in social services and then she relocated to join a community rehabilitation/intermediate care team in Chester. She remained in community services thereafter. Vala's work to date is influenced by her grandmother who lived in Paris until her death in 2005. She embodied the principles of reablement, studying Latvian at the Sorbonne University at eighty, amongst other highly autonomous pursuits. Vala's unwavering quest to explore the experiences of older adults in later life continues today, as a senior lecturer and programme leader in professional education, at the University of Chester.

HAZEL M. CHAPMAN

Dr Hazel M. Chapman is postgraduate tutor at the University of Chester Faculty of Health and Social Care, where she engages with students across all levels of learning. As an adult and learning disabilities nurse, and a Chartered Member of the British Psychological Society, her focus is on person-centred care and person-centred research in health and social care. Her doctoral thesis combined these interests with a study into the experience of health consultations for people with learning disabilities. Her research, with both student nurses and Registered Nurses, into respect in practice has led to the development of new educational approaches within the curriculum. She has also developed new clinical supervision programmes and believes that nurses can only practise person-centred care if they work within a supportive organisation that encourages self-development. Her contribution to this text aims to encourage everyone who wants to learn and achieve their potential.

TIM MANN

The editors are indebted to Tim for providing structure to this project and for keeping us motivated when we started out. Tim qualified as a social worker at Exeter University in 1983, and during his career, worked with both adults and children. He was Assistant Director of Social Services in Cheshire until 2009 when he became Head of Social Work at Chester University. He co-edited *Key Concepts in Social Work Practice* in 2013 (SAGE). Tim is currently an independent 'Fitness to Practise' panel chair for the Nursing and Midwifery Council, a magistrate in both the criminal and family courts, and a trustee of a number of local charities. Throughout his career, Tim has consistently worked with a wide range of other professionals – nurses, Drs, OT's, physio's, speech and language therapists and many others – to achieve the best outcomes for service users. Tim is married with three grown up children.

STELLA ABBINANTE

Stella graduated in 2000. Her nursing career saw her specialise in acute care and cardiology, alongside undertaking various advanced clinical studies to enhance her clinical practice. During this time Stella enjoyed mentoring nursing students which led to her first academic role with a University. As a Senior Lecturer, Stella specialised in skills and simulated led teaching which she developed and led. Stella completed a PGCPD and MSc in Education and presented the results of her Master's thesis Nationally and Internationally. Stella has recently returned to the NHS to support the implementation of the 5 year forward review and Sustainability and Transformation plans. These plans aim to improve health and care in England and represent the biggest National move to join up care in any major western country. In her spare time Stella and her partner Jason enjoy travelling, cooking and socialising with family & friends.

ANNA CLAMPIN

Anna Clampin is a Principal Lecturer and Academic Development Lead for the School of Health Sciences at the University of Central Lancashire and is currently establishing Occupational Therapy provision in the University. Anna is an Occupational Therapist by background and has worked clinically across health and social care sectors and for her professional body (the Royal College of Occupational Therapists), as Head of Education and Learning. During her academic career she has been involved in the development and delivery of education programmes for health and social care professions (particularly allied health). Anna has a particular interested in the professional development of the health and social care workforce across their career.

LISA DIBSDALL

As an experienced occupational therapist, Lisa has dedicated most of her working life to adult social care. She is passionate about interdisciplinary working; recognising that different professions can learn from one another. Lisa's current role is principal occupational therapist (adult care) at Wiltshire Council where she is committed to evidence informed practice and the development of occupational therapists within the organisation. Lisa is currently serving as the social care representative on the Practice Publications Group with the Royal College of Occupational Therapists, commenting on future publications. In addition, she is near completion of PhD research; a qualitative realist study of the role of occupational therapists in reablement services. She is using knowledge gained from her research to support the development of an occupational therapist led reablement service in Wiltshire. Lisa enjoys watching films with her family and paper crafting with friends and is the bandmaster of a brass band.

JACQUI GREENWOOD

After working abroad for a number of years Jacqui qualified as an Occupational Therapist in 2003. Most of her career has been dedicated to working in the community with adults and older adults. Jacqui has been a champion of the benefits of community based reablement services since 2009, being at the heart of the planning, development and then delivery of a Reablement Service in Cheshire. During her specialist practice in stroke rehabilitation, orthopaedics and rapid response, Jacqui has been motivated by the resilience and determination of many of her older clients – proving time and again that a positive attitude and a 'can do approach' can have amazing outcomes. Jacqui is married and has two Jack Russell dogs. After a year blighted by breast cancer, Jacqui's mindset is steadfast: 'never look backwards... you are not going that way'. A good life motto personally and professionally. Occupational therapy is ideally positioned to make this happen.

SUE BINTLEY-BAGOT

Sue Bintley-Bagot is an advanced physiotherapist and owner of a private practice in West Kirby, Wirral. She works with complex patient groups with musculoskeletal problems and offers a personalised and very customised approach to rehabilitation and reablement. Sue is a visiting lecturer at the University of Chester, teaching across a wide range of programmes. She believes in good, precise, diagnostic skills, taking time with her patients to assess thoroughly and to offer patients and families clear education, treatment planning and self management skills. Throughout her career, she has worked with OTs, social workers, dieticians and speech and language therapists, amongst others. When not at work Sue is busy with her three children or out training her cocker spaniel - Lottie. With the odd bit of time that is left, she can be found out running or training, amongst the sand dunes, for her next marathon.

ANNE KEELER

Anne Keeler qualified as a social worker in 1981 and has worked in both children and adults services, including ten years in mental health services. She worked as a Senior Lecturer at the University of Chester for seventeen years where she taught on the BA and MA Social Work, and BA Health and Social Care degrees. Anne has taught a wide range of modules, including Working with Adults and Law and Policy. Anne is married and lives with her husband and two adult sons.

EMMA ROSE-HAYES

Emma qualified as an occupational therapist in 2001 and has been a Senior Lecturer in occupational therapy since 2011. Her career has been varied but has always been strongly grounded in the belief that we promote ability rather than focus on disability. Her special interest is the impact of the environment on occupation, acknowledging the value of accessibility and inclusive design. Effective teamwork features highly on Emma's agenda both professionally, having worked in a range of multi professional teams involving medical staff, allied health professionals and education staff, and personally when taking to the netball court on a cold Saturday in the winter.

GILLIAN WARD

Dr. Gillian Ward is the Research and Development Manager at the Royal College of Occupational Therapists. Prior to this, she was a Reader in Assistive Technologies, Centre for Technology Enabled Health Research at Coventry University. She has a keen interest in the design and usability of assistive technologies to support older people and those with long term health conditions. Gill held a previous appointment at the Health Design and Technology Institute, Coventry University where she led and managed applied research in assistive technologies and provided academic leadership and ethical advice on usability studies of assistive technology products and services. With a successful track record of attracting funding in this area, Gillian has a wide range of research experience including both quantitative and qualitative methods, co-creation and co-design participatory methods. She continues to supervise PhD students as a Visiting Professor to Coventry University.

SUE PHILLIPS

Following her nursing training Sue became a health visitor working mostly in deprived communities. Much of this involved inter-disciplinary working with agencies and a range of health professionals including social services. Sue worked with very vulnerable groups, including for the most part older people, people with long term conditions and those with special needs. After twenty years or so, she needed a change, and moved to education, teaching health and social care professionals. At the University of Chester, she taught a range of programmes, both at undergraduate and postgraduate level. Significantly, Sue was programme leader for a MSc in Professional Studies; a very flexible programme including a range of health and social care professionals. This programme allowed students to learn from other disciplines. Sue retired in 2015, and is now enjoying leisure time, particularly with the Oakland Mavericks, a line dancing group.

FOREWORD

As a practising occupational therapist, working in the field of intermediate care since 2002 and in reablement since 2009, it gives me great
pleasure to introduce this very first book exploring and explaining the
philosophy of reablement. Every chapter delivers a different aspect of reablement and will not only equip you, the reader, with background about
how and why this approach has developed, but will also give you a practical and solid foundation that can be applied in your daily work. Although
this book is aimed at students and support workers, I believe it is essential
reading for all staff members new to the world of reablement.

In addition to experiencing reablement first-hand in my daily job,
I also have the opportunity to see how this approach is being implemented
nationally – through representation of the Royal College of Occupational
Therapists as a member of the National Audit of Intermediate Care steering
group.

As an occupational therapist, I am particularly excited by the philosophy of reablement, as I believe it embodies the core elements of our
training – using a person-centred approach to jointly identify goals that
are meaningful to our clients. Occupations are generally performed in the
most relevant environment for the client – their own homes and local
community. You can probably tell that I am a convert!

I am, however, realistic: although reablement can yield amazing results,
it does not work for everyone. Inevitably some of our clients may choose
not to engage with this approach, and for those individuals with long-term,
progressive conditions the need for ongoing care support will continue,
hence there still remains a place for traditional care.

Barriers may come from clients themselves, from family members and
even from our own staff (Chapter 2). Some clients, especially those who
have previously experienced traditional 'hands-on' care, may decide that
they do not want to be reabled and instead may prefer to be 'cared for'.
Often family members struggle to understand why the reabling staff are
not 'caring for/doing to' their loved one and instead expecting them to
take an active role, 'doing for' themselves. For families living at a distance, it can be reassuring to know that someone will call daily to 'care
for' their relative, and thus they may struggle to take on board the concept of reducing the need for longer term, ongoing care.

Finally, one major barrier I have frequently encountered is from staff themselves – this is also referred to in Chapter 3. Care support staff, who have moved from a traditional care background, may struggle to stand back and encourage clients to 'do' for themselves. There may be feelings of guilt, watching an individual take a long time to perform a task when, with the help of another person, the task could be completed in a fraction of the time. Ah – time! It is challenging to move from a background of only being allocated short time slots to 'do care for' someone and suddenly having to take a step back, fighting the urge to step in and do. Metaphorically keeping one's hands behind one's back takes patience, but it really is a skill worth nurturing. When that 'eureka moment' occurs and the carer sees the look of pride on the client's face as the result of all his/her hard work and achievement, it really is priceless.

For reablement to be effective, a huge cultural change is required by clients, family and staff – this concept is repeated throughout the book. Clear communication is essential. Clients and family need to understand the difference between traditional care and reablement; otherwise misunderstanding will fester and any successes will be short-lived whenever the period of reablement ends. It takes only a few days to learn 'bad habits/behaviours' but several weeks of consistent effort to undo this. Consider perhaps a loved one being admitted to hospital. After only a few days (often wearing hospital gowns/nightwear) they may quickly become 'deskilled' – moving into the role of a patient – no longer performing tasks as they do not feel they have been granted permission to do so.

Last year I underwent some shoulder surgery. The following day I was taken to the bathroom where a perching stool was provided beside the wash hand basin. I accepted that I needed assistance to carry my toiletries into the bathroom but that was when I wanted the help to stop. I automatically filled the wash hand basin and was stunned when the carer reached for my flannel. Indignantly I asked what she was doing and was met with the reply 'I'm going to help you of course'. To her, the most natural thing was to take over, pick up my flannel and attempt to start washing me. I explained that, although I knew I would be slow and most likely struggle to wash with only one functioning arm, I still wanted to do what I could for myself. Bizarrely I felt uncomfortable because it appeared that I had upset the carer by rejecting her help. Just imagine how our clients may feel!

For reablement to work, a clear, consistent and positive approach is required by all team members. If not, do not be surprised if clients receive mixed messages and start to look forward to seeing their 'favourites' who are perceived as more 'caring', rather than other staff who encourage them to become more independent by encouraging them to do for themselves.

For those clients fully aware that the aim of reablement is to achieve meaningful goals, to reduce the need for external care and to 'fly solo', success and independence is something they actively strive for. Consider for yourself, how you feel when you finally achieve something which you have been trying to do for ages. That feeling of success and achievement can be contagious – especially when positively reinforced by others.

For others, success may appear to be a double-edged sword. After weeks of hard work, resulting in achievement of personal and domestic goals, the cessation of visits by reablement staff may be perceived as punishment and social isolation (Petch 2008). Thus, in addition to focusing on personal and domestic care tasks, it is essential to consider social goals – enabling and empowering the client to either return to or become part of their local community.

This book is designed to offer you the opportunity for reflection and consolidation of new learning through exercises and case studies. Although you may already work within a reablement team, each chapter offers a different facet of reablement and will enable you to understand how and why this approach works, leading on to consider future models of service provision and the use of assistive technology with our clients.

Although personally familiar with the theory and practice of reablement, reading this book (Chapter 1) surprised me by making me consider the huge number of informal carers (often with their own health and care needs) who are supporting family members to remain in their own homes. Supporting our growing elderly population while managing care resources is an inevitable 'ticking time bomb'. Something needs to drastically change – this is where the philosophy of reablement can make a radical difference. Excitingly, this approach is dynamic and evolving and is certainly being driven by government agenda. The recently published *NICE Guideline: Intermediate Care including Reablement NG 74* (2017) recommends offering the option of reablement to maximise independence whenever the provision of home care is being considered (1.4.2). The Guideline also recommends the use of positive risk-taking and a person-centred approach to enable clients to learn/relearn new skills and increase their confidence – themes common throughout this book.

Reablement services are growing globally to assist with managing resources and reducing premature dependence on long-term care. By using a reablement approach we can empower our clients; by enabling a 'can-do attitude', focusing on choice and active participation, we can make a lasting difference in their lives. So, as you turn the pages, permit

Valerie Ebrahimi and her colleagues to lead you as you take your next
steps in the world of reablement ...

Cynthia Murphy MSc Dip COT
Chair, Royal College of Occupational Therapists
– Specialist Section Older People
And Senior Occupational Therapist, Rapid Response and Reablement Team
Jersey, December 2017

Reference

PETCH, A. (2008) Re-ablement and the role of the occupational therapist.
Journal of Integrated Care, vol. 16, no. 2, 38–39.

PREFACE

The initial encounter the first editor had with reablement was not in the UK, it was based in Western Australia. At that time, around 2003, Silver Chain, a non-profit home care agency was offering a 'different kind of service'. It encompassed and really seemed to embrace what is considered in health and social care values of independence (here on referred to where possible as autonomy) and choice. Since then the organisation has been the recipient of five awards between the years of 2010 and 2013. The overarching aspect that drew my attention to Silver Chain was their approach to care provision. In fact, as an OT in education, and looking over our original email correspondence, I remember being so intrigued with it that I discussed this with the research development officer within my workplace, a north-west hospital trust. Reablement seemed to me an urgent research priority. I was encouraged to take this interest further. In 2003 working as part of an effective **interdisciplinary** team, in dual roles as community **rehabilitation** therapist and for a **rapid response** service, there was an increasing awareness among us and our managers that services could not sustain the exponential growth. This was not only in terms of the increasing population of older adults, but importantly their future needs. This drive was nonetheless set against another more urgent consideration which was the growing consumer approach to health and social care services. People, our service users, wanted more say in how health and social care services were being run. No doubt this was because of the availability of health information more readily accessible to many through the World Wide Web. Today, in particular, health and social care, alongside its processes and agendas, are no longer a mystery to them. The digital era has made these much more transparent. As a result, health and social care professionals have had to evolve and move towards better partnership working. Now, with the advent of **co-production**, there is a concerted push to more integration, but more importantly better 'ownership' of local community services. This is particularly the case since the devolution of Scotland and Wales but also in relation to moving health care decision making as well as funding to localities (Clinical Commissioning Groups, or CCGs). All this inspired me towards writing a book on reablement – to discover what was out there and how services were being organised and received. I wanted this endeavour to be interdisciplinary, recognising the core skills and values of a wide range of key professionals, namely OTs, social workers, physiotherapists and nurses but essentially the support worker. I also wanted to recognise, and in fact place much greater significance on, the partnership approaches with recipients of reablement and how these individuals might perceive these services.

In considering reablement, there are a number of these services whose core remit is specifically for service users with mental ill health or learning disabilities, and it is important to recognise these. The focus, however, in this book is on older adults. This is for the main reason that reablement services for this group of people are more widely established in the UK and internationally. In addition, most of the co-authors of the chapters work predominantly with this service user group or are involved in the education of students who will be. Despite rapid development in the UK since about 2004, reablement is still a fairly new and often misunderstood service, by those that use it, the service user, their carers and by the public at large. Surprisingly, some health and social care professionals are also not entirely sure about the aims of reablement and whether it works or not. It is not certain either to what extent the subject features in pre-registration programmes for those aspiring to be an OT, social worker, nurse or physiotherapist (PT). To this extent there is somewhat limited literature in terms of research and development as well as policy, although the latter is growing rapidly.

The editors and I hope you find the definitions and range of concepts and debates in this book useful. They are what we and the co-authors for each chapter consider the most important reablement issues, seeking to draw on the successes, as well as areas that raise questions or may be contentious. The aim here is to respond positively but also pragmatically to the increasing levels of need in our communities, as well as rising expectations from people who use health and social care services. There are a number of key themes that emerge in each chapter. You will find that these relate to a greater extent to **person-centredness**, and in some an underlying current suggestive of a **paradigm shift**. This proposed change in thinking is one that encourages a movement from underestimating service user capacity, to one which encourages self-determination.

This textbook is aimed at undergraduate entry-level students and support workers and it is anticipated that they will gain the most from their reading. So, it is our intention to use language that is in current use in practice (the workplace) and at times offer alternatives to this, which are aligned to a change in the way that we need to think about paid care or the issues discussed. Evidently our economy cannot sustain the increasing demand to meet the need for care for older people by maintaining the current arrangements in health and social care – neither at this point in time nor in the future. Collectively and alongside service users, we need to find a way in which to make positive and sustainable changes. These need to take into account the realities of not only limited resources, but a depleting workforce and the physical, psychosocial and financial demands on unpaid carers. Most importantly the views and expectations of those that use health and social care services need to be taken into account and given stronger focus. Co-production is suggested as the means to achieve this. 'We' (all of us with an invested interest in health and social care) need to become more resilient, stop the 'I can't' and move towards a more positive framework of 'let's see how this might work' – together.

ABBREVIATIONS

AAC	Augmentative and Alternative Communication
ADL	Activities of daily living
AT	Alternative Technologies
CCG	Clinical Commissioning Group
COPM	Canadian Occupational Performance Measure
COT	College of Occupational Therapists
CPD	Continuing Professional Development
CSED	Care Services Efficiency Delivery
CSP	Chartered Society of Physiotherapists
CSSR	Council with Social Services Responsibilities
CVA	Cardiovascular accident
DADL	Domestic activities of daily living
DH	Department of Health
ECS	Environmental Control Systems
FACS	Fair Access to Care Services
GP	General Practitioner
IADL	Instrumental activities of daily living
LTC	Long-term condition
MDT	Multi-Disciplinary Team
NHS	National Health Service
NMC	Nursing and Midwifery Council
NSFOP	National Service Framework for Older People
OAT	Occupation, activity and task
OT	Occupational Therapist/occupational therapy
PADL	Personal activities of daily living
PT	Physiotherapist/Physiotherapy
SW	Social Worker
TDP	Telecare Development Programme

INTRODUCTION

Guidance on how to use this book

The book includes eight main chapters, each providing a specific focus. The order of the chapters has been designed to provide a logical continuum of the content, which is intended to build up to a better understanding. Having said this, readers may want to go directly to chapters of interest. Each one has been written separately without specific consideration of the content of others. Therefore, some aspects from one chapter to the next may be repeated, but this is seen as a strength because many of the issues or areas of good practice are important and so we hope that the learning is consolidated.

At the start of each chapter an overview is provided followed by the learning objectives. Each chapter is then divided into sections with subheadings under each of the main headings. Readers may want to go directly to these but it is advised that reading the whole chapter will give greater understanding alongside the context of the discussion. To aid your knowledge and to gain a better view of distinct discussion points, each chapter includes some scenarios. These are based on experiences that practitioners have had in practice, with service user names anonymised and details changed to protect their right to confidentiality. We sincerely thank them for their contributions as they have given us all an insight into their world and the journey that they take in our care. In addition, several student activities and, where relevant, some reflective content, are provided to aid further understanding. Each chapter closes with a summary and some recommended reading. Some terms may not be familiar to you and therefore these have been added to the glossary at the back of the book.

Chapter order and content

The aim of Chapter 1 is to enable readers to grasp and understand the core function and mechanism for change in reablement – occupation, task and activity. First, however, it considers the history associated with reablement services in the UK and how reablement differs from rehabilitation and intermediate care. The debate moves on to whether reablement is a philosophy or simply a method and practical process. The chapter concludes with some of the ethical tensions – such as removing paid care (formal care), the ideas of Ivan Illich in relation to the medicalisation of people and thus turning them into commodities, and the media reaction to issues with the provision of services – to conclude with a real scenario of a failed discharge. Chapter 2 brings a focus to the perspective of the service user and how the policy objectives of reablement can become something that is real for the individual and delivers what they hope for – for themselves. The links between personalisation and person-centred practice are explored, as well as the specific concept of 'co-production' within the reablement process, alongside the importance of 'occupation', cited as the 'vehicle for change'. It is appropriate, then, to move on to a discussion on models of reablement and this is where Chapter 3 takes us: exploring reablement provision to allow all staff involved, as well as service users and their carers, to have an appreciation of what reablement is, what their own particular role may be and what it is trying to achieve. It is only by taking pride in the successes and the outcomes attained, that confidence in the process is nurtured and reablement services can develop further and flourish.

Chapter 4 provides a critical exploration of the concept of dependency and what the essence of independence might be for individuals who may need help at some point in their lives. There is a real danger that support provided by informal carers, as well as by paid staff, can create a state of greater dependency for the person receiving the help, even when the desired outcome of everyone involved is increased independence. The challenge is to move beyond seeing a problem or a need for something to be 'fixed', and to work with the service user and their informal networks of support to identify goals and outcomes and how they can be most effectively realised. Chapter 5 focuses on the role in the reablement process, as we regard them as critical to the delivery of an effective and person-centred reablement service. This is also reflected in our conclusion in Chapter 9. They are the lynchpin in ensuring that people's wishes and aspirations are realised. Support workers are also, at least historically, likely to receive proportionately less training and fewer development opportunities than other professional colleagues involved in rehabilitation and reablement services, and yet crucially are at the 'front end' of the service. Chapter 6 specifically considers the role of reablement for people with long-term conditions (LTCs). These are people who have chronic health problems, and the aim of any intervention is primarily about control and not cure. With 18 million people in the UK affected by LTCs, it is self-evident that this is a key target group for the application of reablement services, both in terms of achieving greater independence for the individuals involved, and as a more effective response to the financial challenge of delivering health and social care services to a growing number of people. The chapter also encourages the further development of interprofessional working from a team perspective to deliver the objectives of reablement services. Chapter 7 seeks to respond to this challenge by considering the concept of self, and how control can be lost as a result of the impact of ageing or an LTC. The key theoretical concepts that support a psychosocial understanding of disability and ageing are explored, as well as the negative impact of stigma on service users. The chapter also discusses the nature and importance of the quality of relationships between service users and all those seeking to help them, including paid staff and informal carers, and how this can have an impact on the eventual outcomes for the service user. Chapter 8 has a specific focus on the contribution of technology to reablement and explores the key ideas for the use of technology to achieve someone's goals and the empowerment of the individual but also the associated tensions such as attention to a potential decrease in human contact. The evidence base for technology is discussed together with examples of how technology can be matched with particular needs of individuals. Finally, the training of health and social care workers in the relevant technology fields is considered, as well as what the future may hold and how the use of technology may be developed further.

Throughout the chapters, and where relevant, reference to research is sometimes necessary, particularly from an evidence-based perspective. At times, therefore, the terminology may be confusing for those new to the subject. Readers are therefore encouraged to look up terms in the glossary or read an introductory textbook on research to gain a better understanding of the subject.

As editors, we have strived to bring together experts in their field to explore the concept of reablement, to encourage the reader to take these ideas into their everyday practice and to continue the journey of improving outcomes for service users. Each co-authored chapter involves at least two authors from different disciplines so as to offer different perspectives on the same topic or concept. There is a tension for some in the idea that reablement is simply a process, with others considering it as an ethos and that there is a need for a paradigm shift in the way in which we all work with those that use our services. The book is aimed, for the most part, at the undergraduate and support worker readership but can serve as an entry point for many others in the field of health and social care. Before turning to Chapter 1, we leave you with this statement from a study by Fine and Glendinning (2005) that describes reablement as '... being able to exercise control over what help is needed'. We suggest capturing this idea in a more sociopolitical context: *the right to self-determination.*

1

Reablement: Shifting Minds

V. Ebrahimi

Chapter outline

To better understand the function and philosophical underpinning of reablement it is essential to have some understanding of the terms Occupation, Activity and Task (OAT). The abbreviation OAT is used from here on when referring to these components collectively.

OAT mechanisms or processes – as applied to practice – are used in reablement interventions to help restore all, or some, aspects of daily living. More often than not restoring this ability to the same level it once was (baseline) can be an unrealistic endeavour; therefore in most instances the aim in reablement is to compensate for this loss. This is achieved by demonstrating to people ways in which to achieve daily living tasks that they may not have experienced in the past, or to undo compensatory methods that are unhelpful. It might include different methods or techniques (for making and transporting a hot drink), to the use of assistive aids (a kettle tipper) and equipment (a perching stool), or by making adaptations to the person's property (a rail fixture or per-manent ramp). In many cases, and before a reablement service starts, people use **compensatory methods** following an impairment (trauma), or from the onset of a long-term condition. Sometimes these are useful and enable a person to continue managing with daily living tasks. Most often, however, these compensatory methods are unhelpful, exacerbating existing functional difficulties, or even causing new previously unrelated ones. Reablement therefore assists in the 'undoing' of unhelpful aspects, relevant to OAT, in the daily lives of older people.

Reablement services and subsequent interventions are often distin-guished by their focus (whether explicit or not) on reducing or prevent-ing paid care input. This focus is prevalent in much of the policy on the subject which supports these types of services. Paid care is what we describe throughout subsequent chapters as regular year-on-year, half-hour to hourly paid support, that is, 'hands-on' help with daily activities. Paid care is often provided by independent agencies contracted by local authorities. In subsequent chapters we refer to this type of support as **formal care**. Aides-memoires for important concepts such as **intermediate care**, relevant theories (the medical and social models) and key words (autonomy) will be provided throughout subsequent chapters.

Reablement can be adjunct or supplementary to intermediate care, but more often than not is provided prior to or following hospital admission. It is not rehabilitation, but is often confused with this type of facilitation, as these interventions also utilise OAT to assist in making positive changes in managing daily living. Another interesting perspective is that reablement is sometimes described by those in the field as a **philosophy** but by many it is seen more from a **pragmatic** level, as a model for practice. To this extent, it is essential to understand the dynamic of formal (paid) care versus **informal care** (includes unpaid partners, relatives, friends and neighbours). This is because both types of care have an important role to play throughout reablement interventions and, in best case examples, when working in co-productivity (**co-production**). We consider these points throughout this book in light of the implications of this for older adults from 50 years of age, but more so for the old old, often but not exclusively identified as 75 years plus. Technology, medical advances and a better awareness of healthy living have pushed up the age at which we generally become frail to a higher level than it was ten years ago.

The way in which OAT is used in reablement is covered very briefly in this chapter. The explanations serve simply to emphasis OAT's centrality in reablement and as a foundation for understanding its importance in reablement interventions. OAT is referred to in one way or another throughout subsequent chapters with examples and scenarios to illustrate the ideas discussed and to enable better understanding. In the first instance, we begin by considering how and when reablement was conceptualised, followed by developments in this contemporary field.

Chapter objectives

This chapter facilitates understanding so that when completed readers will be able to:

➤ Summarise the historical context leading up to reablement in England and to some extent in the devolved countries

➤ Broadly define occupation, activity and task (OAT)

➤ Explain how reablement differs from rehabilitation and intermediate care

➤ Evaluate whether reablement is a philosophy, a new approach to practice or indeed both

➤ Recognise some ethical tensions and dilemmas associated with reablement

The introduction and consequent development of reablement services

The economic reality of formal care

Formal care is clearly one of the greatest financial burdens across the health and social care spectrum. As **local authorities** deal with significant cuts to funding, in recent years the **exponential growth** and demand for social care has risen. Many health trusts are operating at a deficit, warning that this will reach at least 28% by the turn of the decade (a £30 billion funding gap by 2021/22).

In a trade union announcement in 2014, the British Medical Association reported that doctors and medical students were concerned that cuts were 'destabilising a number of GP practices and could lead to their closure' (BMA 2014). This is significant as general practitioners (GPs) who have an understanding of reablement can act as gatekeepers to local services, and those that do not, may do in the future.

In 2006 concerns were raised about the adequacy of social care funding for older people in the long term. Social care is not faring any better than the NHS, with an estimated £4.3 billion shortfall for the same period and a reduction in funding by £3.53 billion (26%). This estimation was made for the latest spending round (LGA & ADASS 2014). In their analysis of the changing patterns to social care provision, the Personal Social Services Research Unit (PSSRU 2013) contended that: 'The scale of reductions in spending and provision [2005/06 to 2012/13] ... are almost certainly without precedent in the history of adult social care' (p. 26).

A year later the *State of the Nation* report (LGA & ADASS 2014) placed further emphasis on this, stating that social care 'has been subjected to draconian cuts as the coalition government has sought to reduce the deficit' (p. 18). This continues under the Conservative administration and who knows where it will lead with more recent changes. In addition to this, the King's Fund (2014a) reported that the reduction in public money spent on social care is creating too much of a demand on individuals and the friends and families who care for them. This demand has caused otherwise moderately healthy and sometimes recently retired individuals to find themselves caring for long hours with little support from services

(Carers UK 2014). Some may have existing long-term conditions which are often exacerbated by stress and tiredness due to managing in an informal caring role; others will acquire them. If we look at the figures for the increasing need for assistance with daily living, a stark picture emerges.

In 2011 there were 800,463 people requiring some form of assistance to help them live independently (Institute of Public Care 2012). Figure 1.1 shows the projected increase from 2015 to 2030 for people aged 65 years and over who will require support at home. It is not clear whether these figures relate to formal or informal care input; however, this is equal to a significant predicted surplus of 293,963 between 2015 and 2030.

The numbers in Figures 1.2 and 1.3 for the same years – between 2015 and 2030 – are particularly high for those who cannot manage domestic (1,657,683) and self-care (1,352,151) tasks autonomously. If we compare the projection by the Institute of Public Care (2012) of those who will require assistance to live independently in 2030 (Figure 1.1) with the numbers in Figures 1.2 and 1.3 – those needing help with specific tasks (domestic and self-care) – it is clear that there is not only a mismatch but the figures are also set to rise significantly. It is also quite likely that many of these domestic or personal care tasks will be carried out by informal carers.

We can assume from Figures 1.1, 1.2 and 1.3 that in the future people will be at an even higher risk of having unmet needs. Another dilemma is that the statistics shown here do not take into account the number of people struggling in our communities who have yet to be identified. The likelihood is that there are many more, extending to possibly over 100,000. This is significant as we know that the impact of care, even at low levels, is often detrimental to the health and well-being of informal carers.

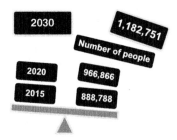

Figure 1.1   Projection for people aged 65 and over helped to live independently

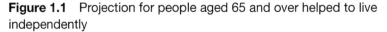

Source: Adapted from the Institute of Public Care (2012)

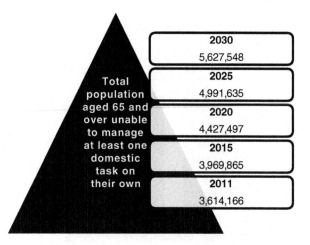

Figure 1.2 People aged 65 and over unable to manage domestic tasks independently

Source: Adapted from the Institute of Public Care (2012)

Two years later, after establishing the level of this need, the Institute of Public Care (2014) published figures for the total population aged 65 and over providing unpaid care. These estimated figures,

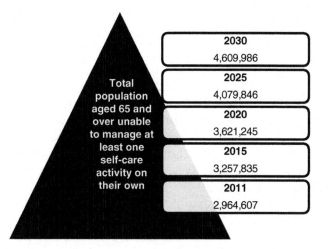

Figure 1.3 People aged 65 and over unable to manage self-care independently

Source: Adapted from the Institute of Public Care (2012)

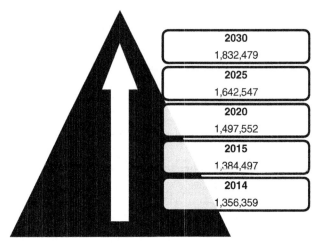

Figure 1.4   People aged 65 and over providing unpaid care to a partner, family member or other person

Source: Adapted from the Institute of Public Care (2014)

based on the 2011 census, are given in Figure 1.4. New figures have been published by the Institute of Public Care (2016) which show trends for 2017 onwards and including 2035. Although there are some differences, the same issues remain with regard to levels of need.

Who cares?

The increase in informal carers by 2030 will be 447,982 (see Figure 1.5), if the year 2015 is taken as a starting point. These carers may themselves require formal care at some point. To illustrate this dynamic more clearly consider the following. The informal carer **'cares for'** their relative/partner/friend/neighbour and over the years may end up requiring formal care themselves. So, to what extent is this a likely outcome? Rather than show all the age ranges and hours we will look at the most significant demographics, those aged 65–69 who make up the bulk of informal carers providing between 1 and 19 hours of care. We also consider those aged 70–85 years and over who will provide care for over 50 hours a week. This is because the greatest concern is with the predictions for over 50 hours of unpaid care per week. As we can see the highest predicted statistic in Figure 1.5 is for the 65–69 age group

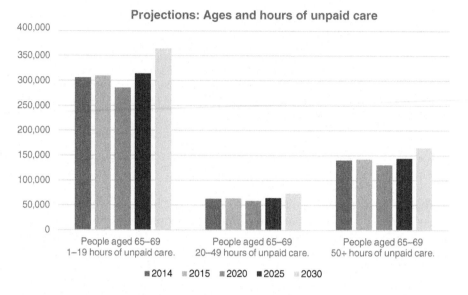

Projections: Ages and hours of unpaid care

People aged 65–69
1–19 hours of unpaid care.

People aged 65–69
20–49 hours of unpaid care.

People aged 65–69
50+ hours of unpaid care.

■ 2014   ■ 2015   ■ 2020   ■ 2025   ■ 2030

Figure 1.5   People aged 65–69 providing unpaid care to a partner, family member or other person

Source: Adapted from the Institute of Public Care (2014)

providing 1–19 hours, but when we compare this to 50 or more hours the figure is very high at 165,252. In addition, and not demonstrated in Figure 1.5, is the rather alarming prediction that, by 2030, 111,699 people over 85 – a 47,366 increase since 2015 – will also be providing this level of care.

The saving to the taxpayer in terms of input by informal carers (as opposed to the average £8 hourly paid rate) is estimated to be approximately in the region of £191 billion per year and over the next five years 106 million people will take on this care role. Many carers do not know that they can claim a carer's allowance (42% approximately) as figures show 1.1 billion of unclaimed allowances each year (Carers UK 2014). This has stark implications because, as mentioned earlier, those aged over 65 years are very likely to need some kind of care later on. Indeed, formal care may even sit alongside their informal caring role. Many informal carers are in the 48–65 age bracket and most often are women. They have jobs or careers and have day-to-day responsibilities – some for school-aged children. There is little or no financial support for these carers. The knock-on effect of this means that many are forced to reduce their working hours, or their career progression may be affected.

FACT 1.1

Almost 4 million of the UK's carers care for 1–19 hours each week. But the numbers caring around the clock, for 50 or more hours each week, are rising faster than the general carer population – an increase of 25% in the last ten years compared to an 11% rise in the total number of carers.

Source: **Carers UK (2014, p. 2)**

These statistics communicate an all-important message which has been echoed time and time again. The number of people requiring formal care in their later years will outstrip available resources. This will create greater demands in the case of hospital admissions, alongside 'bed-blocking', and higher costs for private formal care, as opposed to a universal benefit system. As Beresford (2013) states: 'One of the great strengths of universal benefits is that they create a sense of solidarity and shared understanding. Means tested benefits create the opposite, divisions and misunderstanding.'

The term 'bed-blocking', for those that can or will be able to live autonomously, is used quite frequently in health and social care. It is often seen to be related to a lack of effective co-ordination of care, not reflective of the person, but rather those that are involved in discharge planning at the health end, or in terms of meeting needs in the community. This is often unfair on the services involved because the reality may be that there is a lack of resources, more recently significant staff shortages, or difficulties meeting informal carers' needs in order to support discharge planning. More often than not it only needs one aspect of care provision to fail to cause significant delays. This might be, for example, in setting up a scheme of care in time (formal or **intermediate**), often called a 'care package', or it could be in terms of co-ordination of voluntary services that provide shopping assistance. It may well be an issue with provision of telecare or adaptations required in the person's home. Sometimes a person cannot leave hospital on the basis of needing equipment because there are limited or no family members or neighbours to let providers into the person's home to set it up. The burden of care is even greater when there are informal carers. This is because there is often an expectation (whether explicit or not) to make themselves available, whether to provide access to a property or to accompany their relative home.

Alongside all these issues, acknowledging the person's centrality during their care, as well as their aspirations (as indicated in legislation), will become more and more difficult to achieve. It is even harder to begin to think about the possibilities to combat loneliness through companionship schemes or appropriate group settings. This is where the concept of reablement and a harder drive to find solutions to resource issues can potentially make a significant difference – not only in helping to reduce some of the demands on informal care provision, but also in creating a shift in the way in which we think about **capacity and capability** in the long term.

Student Activity 1.1   Societal responses to ageing and living 'autonomously'

How does society respond to the difficulties people face when living in their own homes? Take a look at the following statements:

'An older person living alone who has no help? ... well they **would have to go** into residential care or a nursing home.'

'We have a responsibility **to look after** older people in our communities.'

The burden of care is demonstrated here as the responsibility of informal carers even if indirectly stated. If people cannot be supported to live at home, is the only solution, then, for formal care (given adequate resources) or institutional living?

How reablement can make a difference

Reablement interventions involve facilitating individuals to learn or relearn activities of daily living (ADL) (DH 2007) following an illness, condition or acquired disability or impairment. These services provide support to people at home following discharge from hospital as well as a means to prevent readmission. For those who have regular **formal care** services, reablement can help in reducing this input completely or partially, but of course occasionally it is found to be inappropriate. Where outcomes are successful, reablement has some cost benefits. Importantly, reablement is supported in Department of Health (DH) social care policy as a preventive initiative that maintains and restores independence (DH 2010a). '**Autonomy**', however, is a more empowering (enabling) term than **independence** and the reason for this is covered in more depth in Chapters 4 and 7. Fundamentally, it is enough to say at this stage that the word 'independent' symbolises, in most cases, the patronising and nega-tive way in which organisations view and refer to people with health and social care-related needs – this is known as **patriarchy**.

The DH (2010a) argument that on completion of a reablement pro-gramme people have significant health improvements in quality of life, in comparison to conventional home care (formal care) (Glendinning et al. 2010), may be true, but wider research is needed to demonstrate if this is indeed the case. There is a greater need to support and justify these assertions if we are to take reablement further forward. At present, how-ever, the problem is that reablement (or the potential for it) is not always immediately apparent to health or social care professionals or those that use these services. This is for several reasons. Consider Scenario 1.1 in light of what you have read so far.

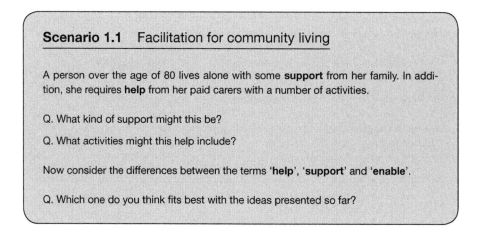

Scenario 1.1   Facilitation for community living

A person over the age of 80 lives alone with some **support** from her family. In addi-tion, she requires **help** from her paid carers with a number of activities.

Q. What kind of support might this be?

Q. What activities might this help include?

Now consider the differences between the terms '**help**', '**support**' and '**enable**'.

Q. Which one do you think fits best with the ideas presented so far?

When reflecting on Scenario 1.1, it becomes clearer that it is not only health and social care services that have created the notion of depend-ence, but society too. Arguably, we all need support and help from time to time. Sometimes, though, we can lapse into stereotyped views of what an older person needs or is capable of. Providing formal care in this way makes people more dependent, when in fact there may be no need for some or even all of this kind of assistance. We need to be more reflective and question our assumptions. With closer scrutiny, this could well be related to professional accountability, the possibility of litiga-tion or involvement in practices which are overly risk-averse. In brief, this means that it is easier to provide formal care alongside adaptations for one ADL alone (justifying that a person is safe) than to contemplate the possibility of complete autonomy. Take, for instance, getting up and down stairs. Providing formal care to assist with breakfast and evening meals may be under the guise of ensuring safety for the person when using a stairlift. However, with practice over time the person could be completely safe carrying out this ADL with no supervision. They might be going up and down stairs several times a day outside of formal contact time. How far do we allow risk in people's lives? It is a waste of resources and costly to the individual, not just in terms of paying for formal carers, but also in its implications on their own sense of well-being: *'I am a danger to myself and need to be very cautious using the stairlift.'* With time, this person can manage the stairlift well by herself (before carer involvement she prepared and cooked her own meals) and has no need for any formal care following reablement. Domestic support could continue once weekly to help with washing, changing the bed linen and some cleaning.

Here we see that the extent of what type of help we provide – or not – becomes critical in reablement. Too often risk aversion prevents people from living their lives autonomously and creates within them a sense of *'I cannot'*, or because someone else is fearful for them it increases their anxiety. We look at this aspect in more depth in Chapter 4. For now, though, take a moment to contemplate what has been said so far in relation to the following statement:

FACT 1.2

'The economic value of the contribution made by carers in the UK is a remarkable £119 billion per year.'

Source: **Carers UK (2011, p. 2)**

Care models

Policy support for reablement typically occurred in 2010 with the advent of government investment to the tune of £70 million (DH 2010b), with more support for social care following in 2012/13 (DH 2011). Further investment resulted when the NHS Commissioning Board transferred funds to local councils in 2013/14 (DH 2012). More recently, the Better Care Fund allocated £3.8 billion in 2015/16 to 'drive closer integration and improve outcomes for patients and service users and carers', with £300 million for Clinical Commissioning Group (CCG) reablement funding (King's Fund 2014a, 2014b). In England joint health and well-being strategies (DH 2013) are moving towards better integration of services across health and social care such as the new Vanguard care models (2016). These are part of the NHS's Five Year Forward plan (DH 2014) with Wirral partners aiming to do this by:

> working much more closely together, commissioning (buying) services jointly, supporting joined-up local services, and working in partnership with the large and diverse local communities and voluntary sector.

> (DH 2014, p. 9)

The notion of integration is not without criticism, however, as historically it has been very difficult to achieve. Yet considerable financial backing to continue developing reablement services is fairly certain. The devolved countries in the UK include Scotland, Wales and Northern Ireland and they have certain powers that are distinct from Westminster parliament in London, England. Although Westminster has reserved powers (the constitution, tax and foreign policy, defence and national security, immigration and citizenship) these do not influence health and social care policy making. The devolved countries, however, share common goals with England: to reduce hospital admissions, reduce the need for paid care and ultimately enable better use of depleting resources. Given this discussion, then, what has led to the increase in people's needs, aside from the oft-quoted statement that this is due to an ageing population?

The exponential rise in social care needs and the aftermath

Forecasts for population expansion were dramatic in the 1990s. Alongside population growth, sedentary lifestyles, a dramatic rise in the consumption of readymade food, smoking and several other social and environmental issues were on the increase. These factors have continued to take their course, negatively affecting health outcomes and giving rise to the increase in long-term health conditions prevalent today. An additional issue is the increase in life expectancy in developing countries. This was cited by Etzioni and colleagues (2003) as the result of technological advances and medical health improvements. Today there are even more advancements, with the ability to extend life across all age groups and for many **acute conditions**. We are now often able to prolong life but there may be a cost to this in terms of subsequent quality of living. There is an awareness that resources are extremely limited. The impact may, then, be seen perhaps on less interaction as **assistive technology** and **telehealth** gain ground.

The idea that technological development benefits humankind is often more celebrated than may in fact be warranted in terms of the issues and threats it imposes. These factors have resulted in the higher numbers of people using health care services in their later years. To add to this is the growing national problem with child obesity (Cole 2006), owing primarily to unhealthier diets and a reduction in exercise as well as more sedentary lifestyles, for example **'gaming'** and using social media, which subsequently also affect adults. Mounting evidence collated in the early part of this century demonstrated that supply would not meet rising health demands unless radical changes were made to health and social care services – models and processes – alongside better use of resources (Buchan and Dal Poz 2002; DH 2000a, 2000b). However, these efficiency improvements may be to the detriment of people's experiences of these services.

Aftermath 1: Limiting resources

FACT 1.3

'In England, continuing with the current model of care will result in the NHS facing a funding gap between projected spending requirements and resources available of around £30bn between 2013/14 and 2020/21 (approximately 22% of projected costs in 2020/21). This estimate is before taking into account any productivity improvements and assumes that the health budget will remain protected in real terms.'

Source: **NHS England (2013, p. 15)**

The debate on 'ineffective [costly] models of care' has been ongoing since the early 2000s (Buchan and Dal Poz 2002; Hyde et al. 2005; DH 2008; Ramesh 2010), with calls for action more recently (NHS England 2013). This is also evident in several government policies: the Francis Report (2013) – prompting policy recommendations – and the Better Care Fund (2014). Models of care refer to any type of service, its process, staffing, allocated resources and location. Over time, many different models have emerged, reablement being one of them, but this results in a consistent drive for evidence of effectiveness. This is often manifest or seen in the targets, or outcomes, that these services are required to meet in order to sustain or justify an increase in funding.

Aftermath 2: Workforce depletion

Another impact on resources is keenly felt in the financing of, and consequent productivity of, the health care workforce (Mackey and Nancarrow 2004; NHS England 2016), a continuous issue since the millennium. In addition to staff shortages – resulting from lack of recruitment, retention and movement, as well as a larger number of retiring employees (DH 2000a; Stanmore and Waterman 2007) – health care professionals continue to be overstretched in the workplace, which impacts on the quality of service provision (Audit Commission 2002; Hewitt et al. 2005). In a report by the King's Fund (2015) the problem is highlighted as particularly significant as services begin work on the Five Year Forward plan (DH 2014). It seems the same issues continue with staffing and morale, and increasing reliance on agency staff is particularly contentious. Following a policy brief prepublication, which included global health workforce labour market projections for 2030, Liu and colleagues (2016, p. 1) found that: 'middle-income countries will face workforce shortages because their demand will exceed supply.' The key issues determine that:

> By 2030, global demand for health workers will rise to 80 million workers, double the current (2013) stock of health workers

> The supply of health workers is expected to reach 65 million over the same period, resulting in a worldwide net shortage of 15 million health workers

> The growth in demand for health workers will be highest among upper middle-income countries, driven by economic and population growth and ageing

The difficulties collectively outlined here are not exclusive to the UK; developed countries within Europe and the USA and Australia also struggle with depleted health care workforces (Buchan and Dal Poz 2002; Bridges and Meyer 2007). Wider international evidence is needed to demonstrate effective models of care. What is discussed here is important for all to consider. It contextualises the global nature of this very serious issue.

"Our greatest asset in reablement: Health care support staff outnumber registered professionals."

It is evident from several sources – historically Davies (2003) and Wanless (2002, 2004) – and identified in statistics from the NHS Information Centre (2009) that health care support staff outnumbered registered professionals in hospital and community settings. The latter data is from 2008. In consideration of a more recent example of unregistered workers in the NHS, the latest statistics for 2014 show a 3.2% rise (11,368) from 357,151 in September 2009 to 362,747 in August 2014.

(For current data, see the Health & Social Care Information Centre website: http://www.hscic.gov.uk/searchcatalogue.) This is positive, and support staff, whether in health or social services, are our greatest asset.

Because face-to-face contact is higher with this staff group, it enables what many consider to be a more 'client-oriented model of service provision'. This was noted by Shield, Enderby and Nancarrow as far back as 2006, but can be argued as equally the case today. In addition, this client-centred orientation is complemented by support workers who are (often) more **generic** in their approach (Nancarrow 2004) alongside having closer focus on interprofessional liaison. This is often seen in intermediate care settings.

The notion of client-centredness: Can we deliver?

In the chapters that follow the theme of person/client-centredness is often referred to. The approach to this type of practice is highly dependent on specific skills such as **active listening**, reasoning and co-partnership as well as the ability to empower the individual. There is often, however, variability in how this is demonstrated in practical terms. This is not due to a lack of interest or attention; more often than not it is because of limited time, staff shortages or inadequate or insufficient training. The potential, however, for developing more person/client-centred relationships is reflected in the effective teaching of, or training in, these skills. We could suppose, too, that higher contact levels between health care support staff and service users will reflect positively in service evaluations and outcomes. Attention to this point is not so apparent in the literature, although the Cavendish Report (2013) is certainly worth scrutiny. This independent review was undertaken following the Mid-Staffordshire crisis and the reported failings in hospitals as well as care homes. The report provides an insight into health care assistants and support workers in the NHS as well as in social care settings. Its central message was that the support workforce has received the least attention up to that point in time in terms of discussions on values, standards and the quality of care in both public sectors. Critically, the development of the support worker role in the UK is given close attention in this book (Chapter 5), alongside other pertinent developments.

The importance of 'actively' working together for improvement: The case for co-production

The prevalence of service user involvement in the development of services (DH 2008, 2010), over the past twenty years, has meant that there is a strong emphasis on 'customer satisfaction' and consultation in government policy. Ocloo and Mathews (2016) contend, however, in their narrative review, that there is a tokenistic approach to supporting patient and public involvement, with progress 'patchy and slow' (p. 626). Co-production has gained increasing interest and momentum and is described by the Social Care Institute for Excellence (SCIE 2013) as 'a meeting of minds coming together to find a shared solution' (p. 7). The power to plan together is mutual, involving both professionals and the general public in delivering support together. There are many definitions and ideas about this new way of working which are discussed in more depth when we examine people's perspectives of reablement in Chapter 2. Importantly, the purchasing power of consumers has also grown significantly in the last decade or so, giving rise to wider consultation and involvement of people who use these services (DH 2006, 2008). In view of this, in the early 2000s new types of worker were considered a viable if not 'cost-effective' option in meeting the exponential rate of increase in demand on NHS services (Wanless 2002, 2004). Some of these relatively new types of worker can now be seen within the field of reablement.

Defining occupation, activity and task (OAT) for reablement interventions

Reablement interventions involve relearning or learning how to carry out ('do') ADL. It is therefore important to define what occupation, activity and tasks are before discussing the practical aspect of reablement any further. Often this learning involves approaching an activity in a different way – sometimes significantly so. From the minute we wake up in the morning to the moment we drift off to sleep at night we are engaged in 'doing'. Closer attention to this is needed given the importance of doing and being able 'to do'. To get you thinking more along these lines take a look at the quotation in Reflection Point 1.1. What is the meaning of this statement?

Reflection Point 1.1 Self-determination: Taking charge and influencing health outcomes

---

'Man, through the use of his hands as they are energized by mind and will, can influence the state of his own health.'

Source: **Reilly (1961, p. 88)**

Reilly's (1961) statement at the Eleanor Clarke Slagle Lecture is a very powerful one. At that time, when medicine dominated health, the idea that a person could influence their own health, rather than manage it solely through medical intervention, was a radical one. It is not so radical today, however, when we take into account public health interventions and the idea of considering the whole person (**holism/holistic**) – which is explicit in much of today's health policy. Without doubt Reilly's (1961) quotation is one of the most famous in occupational therapy (OT) and has been used time and time again to illustrate this pertinent point. Perhaps this is where reablement really comes into its own because we could surmise from this statement that people are experts in activity, in 'doing', in everyday life. But when circumstances change, there may be a need for guidance, while at the same time maintaining control over what we choose to do, when and how we do it.

Student Activity 1.2 Timing and activity

You have an appointment with the doctor at 10am. What are your actions?

List these against the times below:

7.30–7.45	8.15–8.30	9.30–9.45
7.45–8.00	8.30–9.00	9.45–10.00 – In GP waiting area
8.00–8.15	9.00–9.15	

You may have noticed that all these time slots are similar to those that are given to formal carers when working with people in their own homes. Typically, 30 minutes is the minimum.

Q. What is it like to have to be ready to be assisted to get up at 7.30 when you have no morning plans and have slept badly during the night?

'**Doing**' is a verb that typically describes the activities or actions that a person or several individuals engage in. Implicitly, humans affect their world through doing, gaining pleasure and satisfaction through activities, but these also have an internal impact – a personal meaning. In the example above some people might devote at least half an hour to sitting quietly for their breakfast – to reflect on the day ahead. Someone who has a significant change in lifestyle following a stroke might not be able to continue with this routine on this given day, even with the help of a formal carer.

> **Reflection Point 1.2**   A change to your routine
>
> If you had to make a significant change to your routine, what would you be willing to give up?
>
> What would not be acceptable to you?

It is at this point, in the example above, that a reablement intervention can be fraught with tension if the provider is not aware of the personal meaning behind some, or indeed many, of the activities we choose to undertake.

Occupation is the overarching term which embodies activity and task. The most well-known definition of the term is provided by the World Federation of Occupational therapists (WFOT 2016):

> Occupations refer to the everyday activities that people do as individuals, in families and with communities to occupy time and bring meaning and purpose to life. Occupations include things people need to, want to and are expected to do.

Occupation is the central focus for an occupational therapist in their work and they use this therapeutic medium every day. Occupational therapists enable people 'to achieve health, well-being and life satisfaction through participation in occupation' (RCOT 2017).

Activities are primary agents for learning and exploration that occur throughout the human life course. One example of these is domestic activities of daily living (DADL) such as making a cup of tea. We all engage in these DADLs to one extent or another. The 'doing' aspect of an activity occurs within and during growth and development. Engagement in any given occupation is a part of being human; the intrinsic value of this is argued throughout the chapters in this book. It is a vehicle for healing and well-being. The Peter Principle (1960) argues that: 'Competence, like truth, beauty, and contact lenses, is in the eye of the beholder' (Peter and Hull 2009, p. 32). What may be considered as an activity completed well (competently) could be the opposite to someone else's idea of competence or capability. This poignant statement on competence is revisited in Chapter 2. Competence is the mechanism in which the person who uses health and social care services will be assessed on (or judged) when carrying out any ADLs. It therefore has great significance. Let us take the following as an example to illustrate this point. We will do this in the context of an occupation which is observed or concomitant in quite a few reablement interventions: making tea.

Tea drinking has been somewhat embedded in the British way of life, both historically and from a social perspective, even if the great caffè latte seems to be taking precedence. Similarly, in other cultures there is an 'attached' symbolic meaning to sharing tea or a coffee – comfort, friendship, respect and support. If we consider the actions associated with tea- or coffee-making, such as patterns of voluntary movement, positioning of the body, **cognitive** processing and **perception**, these can be associated with the tasks one needs to undertake.

Tasks need to be completed in order to make a cup of tea with the making of tea as the **activity** itself. A visual perspective of how this might work is provided in the Figure 1.6. This systems process diagram is divided into three sections showing input, process and output.

Reflection Point 1.3   When making tea which tasks would you say are mostly cognitive?

You might say 'all of them!' and you would be right, but after a life of tea-making are we really thinking about it? What part of it is just automatic?

When faced with an impairment in function what happens next – do we overthink?

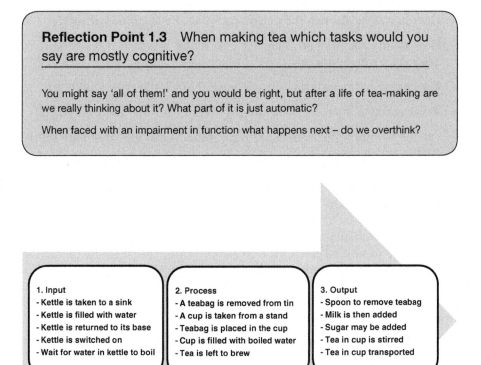

Figure 1.6   A basic activity analysis: Possible process and order of tasks when making a cup of tea

When considering these aspects, we can take it even further but then the elements in the flow chart will change. Look at Reflection Point 1.3 and then see if you can apply the examples in Figure 1.6.

Of course Figure 1.6 is a very simplistic overview, as many other important factors need consideration, such as culture, which means the tea might be made differently or the items and utensils used may vary. Motor processes, such as voluntary movement, positioning and cognitive processing, all play a major part and do not feature in this diagram. Neither does the environment in which the activity takes place nor the aids and possible adaptations. What this process does illustrate is some of the issues that arise when we consider an older person with long-term health needs, disability and/or impairment.

Questions that might arise include:

> How much weight can the person carry? (1. Kettle filled with water)

> How steady are they on their feet? (1. Kettle is returned to its base; 3. Tea in cup transported)

> How good is fine motor control (fingers)? (1. Kettle is switched on)

> What is the tolerance for standing? (1. Wait for water in kettle to boil)

> Are they aware of their surroundings (home)? (2. Where items are kept)

> How steady are their hands? (2. Cup is filled with boiled water)

> What is their short-term memory like? (1. Wait for water in kettle to boil; 2. Tea is left to brew)

Although these issues have been covered in very scant depth here, they do illustrate some real tensions that people can experience in the act of *'doing'*. This leads to some further questions for refection:

> Can we underestimate or make prejudgements about an older person's skills?

> If so, does this lead to more dependence on formal care than is necessary or needed?

> Likewise, can we overestimate ability, leading to involvement in tasks that are beyond the person's capability?

Let us now consider the aims of other types of services, like reablement, that help restore, maintain or compensate for, and essentially facilitate people in carrying out daily activities. This is necessary because these

Reflection Point 1.4   Improving functional mobility and self-care

Research carried out by Lewin and Vandermeulen (2010) showed an improvement in functional mobility following reablement, and improvements in self-care were found by Lewin and colleagues in 2013.

Q. Think about which particular factors may have influenced the positive outcomes of both studies. Write down three possible influences and then access the following links to see the results:

Lewin and Vandermeulen (2010) study: http://www.ncbi.nlm.nih.gov/pubmed/19674125

Lewin, Alfonso and Alan (2013) study: http://www.ncbi.nlm.nih.gov/pubmed/24124354

services can be an adjunct towards the referral to a reablement service. To do this it is important to go back to the start of the 21st century. This will help to contextualise how the need to address shortfalls in older care provision came about.

Rehabilitation and intermediate care: Different or the same?

Public health strategies have been criticised in the past for failing to recognise wider environmental and social factors that contribute to health and well-being (Age Concern 1999; Age UK 2014a; Davidson 2014). Furthermore, resource pressures as well as community reforms meant that older people were receiving services only when their needs had become acute (DH 1999; DH 2001). One of the recommendations, therefore, by the National Service Framework (NSF) in 2001 was significant investment in prevention and rehabilitation. The amount projected for 2003/04 for intermediate care was £900 million (DH 2000b). In 2005 the then Health Secretary John Reid announced that a £135 billion investment in the NHS would be allocated to English Primary Care Trusts for the two financial years 2006/07 and 2007/08. He stated that the money would ensure that there would be greater support for people with long-term conditions closer to home (DH 2005). In 2006/07, £64.3 billion was allocated and £70.4 billion in 2007/08; however, it is not clear how much of this budget was specifically allocated to intermediate care services. (For information on current funding for 2016/17, see https://www.

england.nhs.uk/ourwork/part-rel/transformation-fund/bcf-plan/.) The Better Care Fund Allocations are reported for each locality as a whole but do not refer specifically to figures for intermediate care as this is for the CCGs to determine independently.

Intermediate care follows the principles of rehabilitative strategies or interventions, which seek to restore, maintain or compensate for residual disability or a long-term condition or impairment. The difference here is in location and specificity in terms of, for example, ongoing work to enable better functioning of upper body movement following hospital discharge. While rehabilitation takes place in acute hospital settings, in the community (people's homes) or within specific organisations such as Headley Court (injured veterans of the armed forces), intermediate care has a somewhat different focus:

➢ It has a specific age intake of usually those who are aged 60 and over (variations across the UK)

➢ It is located within nursing homes (contracted beds) or specific community-based facilities

Or:

➢ It can be based in a person's home such as in the case of reablement (hospital at home/following a rapid response service)

➢ It involves referral from GPs/other professionals, **rapid response** or at point of hospital discharge

Although the stipulation for intermediate care came with a proviso that it is for anyone over the age of 18, generally speaking these services cater for older adults over 60. Services are predominantly located in community hospitals (41%) followed by standalone facilities (13%) and nursing homes (no data) (NAIC 2013). This involves a limited, no-charge stay, much like reablement, of generally up to six weeks (variations across the UK) with charges applying thereafter.

When referred to an intermediate care facility, each person is generally provided with a room and an en-suite bathroom. They have regular daily contact with nurses to assess that they continue to be medically stable; they will probably see an OT and physiotherapist (PT) as well, and in varying degrees. There are several routes to access intermediate care services, but all potential routes into the service require the person to be medically sound with some accepting those with dementia or other cognitive-related conditions. Referral routes can come via the GP, as a 'step down' following hospital discharge or as a result of a breakdown in coping strategies in the community, sometimes known as hospital at home. The difference from rehabilitation in the context of intermediate care is that rehabilitative interventions and services seek to help people recover function. Reablement, on the other hand, aims to help accommodate illness or disability by learning or relearning ADL importantly in the person's own home, often but not exclusively via a reduction or removal in formal care.

In the instances of long-term conditions, for example, energy conservation techniques may be taught when an older adult has debilitating arthritis. By the term debilitating, we mean affecting the quality of life (pain and restricted movement) and daily living (activities and associated tasks). Rehabilitation focuses on making improvements in function generally and may involve adaptations or equipment to assist with this. In the instance of a person with arthritis, one of his or her goals may be to be able to brush their teeth unassisted. This might then involve provision of a perching stool and some putty to enlarge the handle of the toothbrush. The adjustable height and slanted seat on the stool helps to reduce fatigue and takes some of the weight off the person's large joints (knees) while still encouraging muscular activity in the legs. The enlarged toothbrush enables a better grip when there is limited strength and movement but it also relieves and prevents pain and exacerbation. Of course, a similar course of action might occur in reablement. In that context, however, not only is the aim to enable a person with a number of tasks of daily living, but it may also be to reduce or cease formal care – helping a person on towards as much autonomy as possible and with a preventative focus. Reablement always takes place in a person's home and this is a key difference as well as the length of time. Specific interventions common to reablement services are covered in more depth in Chapter 5, which also examines the essential role of support workers.

Since the introduction of intermediate care and other related community services in 2001, there has certainly been a significant reduction in delayed discharges from acute hospitals. This reduction was 64% up to 2005 and equated to a release in beds of 1.5 million (DH 2006). On the other hand, this positive data is not so evident for intermediate care four years later following a review by Woodford and George (2010). They appraised the impact of a range of intermediate care services on freeing up acute hospital resources for people with a variety of medical conditions. The evidence, however, was found to be weak with no reliable data to suggest that acute hospital use is reduced and indeed that costs could increase. The National Audit of Intermediate Care (NAIC) in 2012/13 found that 20% of bed-based services had a waiting time of about four days or more, with two-thirds waiting in acute beds (NAIC 2013). In addition, access from emergency admissions to intermediate care was not routine. In the same report it was established that 61% of people completing reablement had no ongoing home care needs. A more recent report by NAIC (2015, p. 3) offers a far more positive perspective and includes reablement under the Intermediate Care umbrella. It concludes that: 'the four service models included in the audit (crisis response; home based; bed based; and re-ablement) deliver good outcomes.'

Despite the reported success of reablement, the NHS as a whole is in crisis, with a workforce that continually struggles in their delivery of quality services. Funding to meet the demands and hopes of an ageing population continues to present significant political and structural challenges even without the added impact and consequence of stringent and restrictive economies. The search for more effective models of care also continues.

FACT 1.4 The effectiveness of intermediate care and reablement – 2015

The overall results for NAIC (2015, pp. 52–53) showed a high level of positive outcomes for service users: 92% of people maintained or improved their dependency score in both home-based and reablement services (in NAIC 2014 the figure was 92% for home-based services). In bed-based intermediate care, 93% of people maintained or improved their dependency score (94% in NAIC 2014).

Perhaps counter-intuitively, the results (NAIC 2015, p. 53: tables 6.1–6.9) suggest that people starting reablement are more dependent than those starting home-based intermediate care services.

It seems that goal attainment levels were not good for those using a reablement service and for some respondents this was due to a lack of goal setting. When asked the question given in Table 1.1, the following answers were provided in a questionnaire returned by 8,372 people.

Table 1.1 Have the intermediate care goals set on admission for the service user been achieved?

Intermediate care service	Yes	No	Partially	Goals not set on admission
Home-based	72%	5%	16%	7%
Bed-based	77%	6%	14%	2%
Reablement	53%	9%	21%	17%

Source: NAIC, (2015, p. 53)

It is important to note here that there were fewer respondents to reablement services in the return of the questionnaire (1,692) compared to home-based (4,233) and bed-based (2,877). So this data needs to be interpreted with caution. Goal setting is discussed in more depth in Chapters 3 and 5.

Ethical tensions and dilemmas associated with the provision of reablement

Traditionalist ideas suggest that as we reach older adulthood we become less interested in being active and that we choose to withdraw from many activities and connections. This requires some thought, however, as such assumptions for the most part are inaccurate and do not provide a true picture. Certainly, when health is compromised or a person develops a long-term condition, they are likely to want to take things more slowly; but is this not the case for everyone – regardless of age? To some extent (and although this statement may bear some truth in certain situations) when a person deteriorates, for example with their mobility, it is more often due to a *lack of effective consideration of individual situations and subsequent input – or lack of*. This may be due to isolation and/or no significant other to support the person. There is no doubt that health and social care professionals and support workers are often overstretched. This is in part due to absences in the workplace, which are often a consequence of either recruitment issues (lack of funding) and/or retention issues (a high level of mobility and an ageing workforce). Added to this is the exponential growth of people requiring an array of services. Age UK (2015) illustrate this well in their statement that: 'the over-60s is the fastest-growing group in society … ageing is not an illness, but it can be challenging.'

Restlessness, loneliness and isolation are often seen in many of these situations, perhaps resulting from not having access to local community information, or not knowing how to go about setting up additional support outside of the NHS or social care services. This additional support, however, can be tailored to particular preferences – for example, horticulture, film appreciation clubs or simple gatherings where people can meet and chat. This is in stark contrast to day centres. To this effect reablement can make a difference, but not if we solely focus on personal care needs over social ones. We must make a concerted move forward to address this very important aspect of *'being and connectedness'*. It is not a question of having to provide specific opportunities in reablement, but encouraging and facilitating people to reach a social goal is likely to motivate far more than sole focus on personal activities of daily living (PADL) and DADL.

Although there is no great desire here to enter into too strong a debate on social iatrogenisis, it is nonetheless important to understand the idea. **Social iatrogenesis** was first described by the Russian Ivan Illich who died in 2004. In his discussion of Illich's provocative ideas, Barnet (2003) explains that a number of types of iatrogenesis exist – social and structural. The term iatrogenesis itself refers broadly speaking to the problems medicine and those affiliated to it create, through clinical misjudgement or neglect, incorrect diagnosis and to hospital-induced disease or injury. Social iatrogenesis refers to the dependence on medical expertise which leads to the medicalisation of life. An example of this is our frequent use of antibacterial sanitising gel and access to store-bought blood pressure monitors for use in the home. This turns people into commodities through the 'selling of health'. **Structural iatrogenesis** similarly places dependence on medical intervention through the sanitisation and technological replacement of coping – for example, with birth and death. There are, of course, as with any proposed ideas, critiques of Illich's concept, but clearly people have become very dependent, reliant and almost accepting of these influences. The professions of social work, nursing, youth and community work and so on, are all historically part of what can be seen as a 'pseudo-medical' form of professionalism. This is inevitable but by being aware of our influence – our power – we can move on to something much more positive long term and this is where empowerment takes more of a central focus.

Oftentimes there is an assumption or view that *older people automatically disengage from society* – or should do so. In many instances, it is even implicitly encouraged by some people or seen as natural. Books have been written about the notion that older people should prepare for 'disengaging'. This idea is taken further in Chapter 7 when disengagement theory is contrasted with the more positive gerotranscendence. Both offer different perceptions of what happens when a person retires and/or reaches 'old age'. Gerotranscendence, however, offers a more individualistic perspective than the concept of disengagement. Yet what is clear is that even today individualism is not really addressed in full by health and social care staff, as we will see to some extent in the discussion on socialisation in Chapter 3. The idea Thursz, Nusberg and Prather (1995) presented in the mid-1990s remains one that is today easily recognised:

> Older people are one of the last groups with which the notion of empowerment has become associated. Yet the 'privileges' it represents – the ability to make informed choices, exercise influence, continue to make contributions in a variety of settings, and take advantage of services – are critically important to the well-being of elders (p. ix).

There is a need to relinquish existing traditionalist ideas about *how we should age*, including the glamorised ideas about what successful ageing is – running marathons or modelling in high-profile magazines. This is an individual perception and not one that is catch-all. Health and social care practitioners, whether professional registrants or in a support role, need to be aware of how people (Society in general) perceive competence. These perceptions might differ drastically from those involved in the provision of reablement interventions.

Despite public health initiatives to improve hospital admissions, it is clear that resources are overstretched and this is going to get worse, not better. It is an area of contention in the public domain which is often reflected in the media:

FACT 1.5

Typical headlines in national newspapers or online forums:

'Outrage over online bids for elderly care home contracts'

(RT Question More, March 2015)

'A million elderly people lack basic social care as unprecedented funding cuts leave struggling NHS to pick up the pieces'

(The Independent, April 2015)

RT Question More (2015) provides news forums, with some stating in their debate on care that a system of auction to deliver the lowest cost provision of care moves away from personalisation. The second example in Fact 1.5 is taken from *The Independent* newspaper, in which, in the same year, social care was criticised as new figures from Age UK suggested that over a million older people are not getting their care needs met at home. In addition, a number of people, due to delays in hospital discharge, return home in a far worse position than they should. Many older adults are discharged either too early or inappropriately to intermediate care settings to steadily become more and more vulnerable. These individuals are at greater risk of ending their lives in a nursing home. Scenario 1.2 is taken from one such situation which is all too common across health and social care services; it is as shocking as it is saddening.

Scenario 1.2   When health and social care services fail

Social and medical history

Barbara is a woman of 75 living alone in a third-floor apartment in a northern city centre. Although having moved from London in 2010 to much better accommodation, she felt rather isolated in her new community. Barbara joined a group called 'Companions' which she found for herself. She very much enjoyed this compared to previous meetings held by the 'University of the Third Age' (U3A).

Following a **subarachnoid haemorrhage** in 2001 Barbara often experienced exacerbations of tiredness, visual disturbance (which did self-correct) and initially rather serious **agoraphobia**. To date she also has some difficulties with cognitive processing which results in the use of quite a lot of note-taking and listing of chores and bills she needs to attend to. This activity, however, helps her and despite having a transient ischemic attack in 2014 she was doing very well and was autonomous in all ADL and DADL. Her daughter was not involved in supporting any of Barbara's ADL. Occasionally they would go to restaurants and movies and away on occasional weekend trips together.

Event leading to hospital admission

Around the end of November 2015 Barbara had a fall resulting in a right hip fracture. She was taken to Accident and Emergency (A&E). While there, a profiling bed including an airflow mattress was provided. Barbara's sutures (staples/stitches), and the wound, was healing well following surgery to fit a dynamic hip screw (DHS). The intention was to discharge her for reablement as this was considered appropriate for her situation and ability. Throughout the time prior to the discharge Barbara either sat in a high chair or lay in bed. Hardly any rehabilitation, took place across the 11 days she stayed on the specific hip fracture ward despite two visits from an OT support worker, one from an OT and visits every other day from a PT. Barbara had to wait for almost a week for an airflow mattress to be delivered to the intermediate care unit. She could have potentially left a week earlier if this had not been an issue.

Discharge to a 'reablement' facility

It was explained to Barbara's daughter that the place she was going to would be rehabilitative and was referred to as a reablement service. She would get an opportunity to build up her confidence, mobility and PADL while there. This was not discussed with Barbara. It turned out, however, that she had been discharged for 'short term care and support' in a care home. This did not come to light until much later. Her daughter was not able to monitor Barbara's care as a result of a serious lung infection requiring urgent hospital care.

During Barbara's eight-week stay she only moved from one of two living room chairs to eat or to go to bed. Her experience on the mattress at night was painful and she could not sleep, often lying awake most of the night. When Barbara asked on numerous occasions to have it replaced with a standard mattress, her requests were often met with a nod but no further action was taken. Several of the other individuals had dementia or Alzheimer's disease. Barbara had no option but to sit in the allocated

▶

◀

living room with earplugs as the television was kept on 24 hours a day. The larger quieter main living room seemed to be used only by staff or for group activities. These group activities were always seated and during her time in the care home Barbara had three visits from a PT, the latter two towards the end of her stay and one or two from an OT. Barbara carried out the PT exercises provided religiously at the start of her stay but complained when, by the fourth week, she was still doing the same ones. No clear therapy goals were identified to Barbara by anyone or when her daughter made enquiries following her own discharge from hospital.

Discharge home

On discharge home Barbara had chronic back pain. When standing she leaned to her left side (possible **kyphosis**) and walked very cautiously with a walking stick. The tiredness was much worse and after half an hour she often had to sit down. In addition, she had post-operative oedema in the right leg and later it transpired that this was most likely because of the lack of mobility and PT and OT input, including appropriate involvement of the 'care home' staff. Barbara experienced pain all the time, when standing, lying down and sitting. Given that she had surgery for a hip fracture and that this was almost three months later, this is unusual. It is likely this is related to the immobility and static seated posture throughout her stay. The PT and OT visited twice in the community and then withdrew. Barbara was provided with a three-wheeled Delta Walker and a walking stick. She practised with the PT walking 20 metres to a local newsagent but no further.

Subsequently, a private PT was engaged by Barbara as she had so many concerns about the changes to her posture, the exacerbated tiredness and pain. The PT advised Barbara immediately to move off the prescribed walking stick to a four-wheeled walker. This had a carry bag at the front and enabled her to walk with more confidence. It also allowed Barbara to practise standing more upright – but safely! Her daughter continues today to assist with shopping, and because at present Barbara has so much pain her opportunity to socialise is greatly diminished. Barbara and her daughter meet once a week for cocktails and a chat.

A year post-discharge Barbara was so frustrated and angered by the experience that she took the matter to Healthwatch Advocacy.

Reflection Point 1.5 Defending choices: The importance of clarity in communication and subsequent action/s

Some of the recommendations from this scenario are puzzling:

1. Why was there a need for an airflow mattress? There seemed to be no risk to skin integrity so was the above equipment used because the referral was inappropriate?

2. If an individual is complaining of pain using a prescribed mattress, would it not be appropriate then to have this properly assessed?

3. What is the rationale of leaving someone to be seated at intervals of two hours and for a period extending over ten hours?

▶

◀

4. Why was Barbara referred to a care home rather than reablement or intermedi-ate care, when clearly she was medically stable with no skin integrity issues, fully autonomous in ADLs prior to the fracture and her mobility was good?

5. More importantly, why was she not told about the discharge plans? Her daughter was told that she was being referred to a reablement service but clearly it was a care home.

Basic communication should never be so bad that individuals leave a service worse off or depressed, as in this scenario. Despite the stretched resources in health ser-vices (both financial and in terms of staffing) we can at least communicate intentions clearly and consistently – even if sometimes these do not meet the expectations of the person.

Even if there is a possibility that a place at another more appropriate facility becomes available, is it right to refer someone from hospital to a service which does not meet a person's needs or their expectations?

We thank Barbara for sharing her story, who at the time of publishing, asked not to be anonymised or given a **pseudonym**. We had to nonetheless for obvious confidentiality reasons. Barbara said that providing a picture of her recent experience was a matter of importance to her, and that students and support workers should know about the issues associated with a failed discharge. She understood the issues with staffing and resources but felt that she had been badly treated overall. Scenario 1.2 highlights several issues and illustrates another from the earlier statement, regarding how millions of informal carers go unpaid (see Fact 1.2). Most carers have no choice in these situations, with many juggling complex family lives, careers and finan-cial issues. Often this is because they do not meet the criteria for a Carer's Allowance which was £61.35 per week in 2014/15 (Age UK 2014b) or they are over the threshold allowance. The evidence, that these carers suffer stress and new or exacerbated health conditions later in life, is extensive and con-tinues to increase year by year (Carers UK 2011, 2014).

Summary

➢ The term reablement has been around in the UK since around 2004.

➢ The principles of this type of service provision are not new. They have been inte-gral to the core practice and values of OT since the First World War.

➢ Informal carers save the economy billions but their health and well-being are at risk if their concerns are not adequately addressed.

▶

◄

➢ Intermediate care and rehabilitation employ some of the same techniques but the approach and long-term objectives are different.

➢ Addressing workforce shortages, appropriate use of agency staff and more effective and far-reaching training opportunities are critical for more lasting change.

➢ There is a continuing need to challenge the stereotypes and negative perceptions of what older people can or cannot do. These views are held not only by the public, but also by the health and social care workforce at large.

Recommended reading

HAMMEL, K. W. (2006) *Perspectives on disability and rehabilitation: Contesting assumptions; challenging* practice. Edinburgh: Churchill Livingstone.
HEALTH AND SOCIAL CARE INFORMATION CENTRE. (2016) *Data Catalogue.* Available at: http://www.hscic.gov.uk/searchcatalogue (Accessed 10 June 2015).

References

AGE CONCERN. (1999) *The future of health and care for older people: The best is yet to come.* London: Age Concern. (Debate of the Age – The Millennium Papers).

AGE UK. (2014a) *Loneliness a 'serious issue' for older people.* Available at: http://www.ageuk.org.uk/latest-news/archive/loneliness-and-isolation-a-serious-issue-for-older-people-/ (Accessed 12 February 2015).

AGE UK. (2014b) *Carer's Allowance.* Factsheet No. 55. Available at: http://www.ageuk.org.uk/brandpartnerglobal/gloucestershirevpp/factsheets/carers/carer's_allowance_fcs.pdf (Accessed 3 June 2015).

AGE UK. (2015) *Who are we.* Available at: http://www.ageuk.org.uk/about-us/who-we-are-/ (Accessed 12 February 2015).

AUDIT COMMISSION. (2002) *Recruitment and retention: A public service workforce in the twenty-first century.* Public sector national report. London: Audit Commission.

BARNET, R. (2003) Ivan Illich and the nemesis of medicine. *Medicine, Health Care and Philosophy,* vol. 6, no. 3, 273–286. DOI:10.1023/a:1025991708888.

BERESFORD, P. (2013) Why means-testing benefits is not efficient or fair. *The Guardian,* 14 January. Available at: https://www.theguardian.com/social-care-network/2013/jan/14/means-testing-benefits-not-efficient-fair (Accessed 11 February 2015).

BETTER CARE FUND. (2014) *Better Care Fund*. Policy framework. Available at: https://www.gov.uk/government/uploads/system/uploads/attachment_data/file/381848/BCF.pdf (Accessed 10 June 2015).

BMA (BRITISH MEDICAL ASSOCIATION). (2014) *'Bid to halt general practice funding cuts'*... Available at: https://www.bma.org.uk/news/2014/june/bid-to-halt-general-practice-funding-cuts (Accessed 25 November 2017).

BRIDGES, J. & MEYER, J. (2007) Policy on new workforce roles: A discussion paper. *International Journal of Nursing Studies*, vol. 44, no. 4, 635–644. DOI: 10.1016/j.ijnurstu.2006.08.008.

BUCHAN, J., & DAL POZ, M. R. (2002) Skill mix in the health care workforce: Reviewing the evidence. *Bulletin of the World Health Organization*, vol. 80, no. 7, 575–580.

CARE QUALITY COMMISSION. (2011) *The state of health care and adult social care in England 2010–2011*. Available at: http://www.cqc.org.uk/sites/default/files/media/documents/state_of_care_2010_11.pdf (Accessed 2 February 2014).

CARERS UK. (2011) *Valuing Carers 2011: Calculating the value of carer's support.* Available at: http://circle.leeds.ac.uk/files/2012/08/110512-circle-carers-uk-valuing-carers.pdf (Accessed 20 January 2014).

CARERS UK. (2014) *Facts about carers*. Policy Briefing. Available at: http://www.carersuk.org/for-professionals/policy/policy-library/facts-about-carers-2014 (Accessed 2 February 2014).

CAVENDISH REPORT. (2013) *The Cavendish Review: An independent review into healthcare assistants and support workers in the NHS and social care settings.* Available at: https://www.gov.uk/government/uploads/system/uploads/attachment_data/file/236212/Cavendish_Review.pdf (Accessed 16 September 2016).

COLE, T. J. (2006) *Early causes of child obesity and implications for prevention.* 2nd Scandinavian Paediatric Obesity Conference. Available at: http://www.ucl.ac.uk/paediatric-epidemiology/pdfs/Acta_Paed_2007_(P048).pdf (Accessed 3 May 2010).

RCOT (ROYAL COLLEGE OF OCCUPATIONAL THERAPISTS). (2017) *Live life your way.* Available at: https://stage2.cot.co.uk (Accessed 25 November 2017).

DAVIDSON, S. (2014) *Evidence review: Loneliness in later life*. Age UK. Available at: http://www.ageuk.org.uk/professional-resources-home/knowledge-hub-evidence-statistics/evidence-reviews/ (Accessed 7 September 2014).

DAVIES, C. (ed.). (2003) *The future health workforce*. Basingstoke: Palgrave Macmillan.

DH (DEPARTMENT OF HEALTH). (1999) *Promoting independence: Preventative strategies and support for older people*. Report of the SSI Study. London: Department of Health.

DH (DEPARTMENT OF HEALTH). (2000a) *Meeting the challenge: A strategy for the allied health professions*. London: DH. Available at: http://webarchive.nationalarchives.gov.uk/+/www.dh.gov.uk/assetRoot/04/05/51/80/04055180.pdf (Accessed 20 November 2017).

DH (DEPARTMENT OF HEALTH). (2000b) *The NHS plan: A plan for investment, a plan for reform*. Command paper: 4818-I. London: HMSO. Available at: http://webarchive.nationalarchives.gov.uk/+/http://www.dh.gov.uk/en/

Publicationsandstatistics/Publications/PublicationsPolicyAndGuidance/
DH_4002960 (Accessed 25 November 2017).

DH (DEPARTMENT OF HEALTH). (2001) *National Service Framework for Older People*. London: DH.

DH (DEPARTMENT OF HEALTH). (2005) £135 *billion investment to improve to NHS services and health of the nation*. Press Release No. 2005/0050. London: DH. Available at: http://www.dh.gov.uk/PublicationsAndStatistics/ PressReleases/Press (Accessed 15 November 2006).

DH (DEPARTMENT OF HEALTH). (2006) *Our health, Our care, Our say: A new direction for community services*. London: DH. Available at: https://www.gov. uk/government/uploads/system/uploads/attachment_data/file/272238/6737. pdf (Accessed January 2018).

DH (DEPARTMENT OF HEALTH). (2007) *Putting people first: A shared vision and commitment to the transformation of adult social care*. Ministerial concordat. Available at: http://www.dh.gov.uk/en/Publicationsandstatistics/ Publications/PublicationsPolicyAndGuidance/DH_081118 (Accessed 11 June 2014).

DH (DEPARTMENT OF HEALTH). (2008) *High quality care for all: The NHS next stage review final report*. London: DH. Available at: http://www.dh.gov.uk/ prod_consum_dh/groups/dh_digitalassets/@dh@en/documents/digitalasset/ dh_085828.pdf (Accessed 10 February 2009).

DH (DEPARTMENT OF HEALTH). (2010a) *A vision for adult social care: Capable communities and active citizens*. Social Care Policy. London: DH. Available at: http://www.dh.gov.uk/prod_consum_dh/groups/dh_digitalassets/@dh/@en/@ ps/documents/digitalasset/dh_121971.pdf (Accessed 2 February 2013).

DH (DEPARTMENT OF HEALTH). (2010b) *The operating framework for the NHS in England 2011–12*. Policy Paper. Available at: https://www.gov.uk/government/ publications/the-operating-framework-for-the-nhs-in-england-2011-12 (Accessed 11 June 2014).

DH (DEPARTMENT OF HEALTH). (2011) *The operating framework for the NHS in England 2012–13*. Policy Paper. London: DH. Available at: https://www. gov.uk/government/publications/the-operating-framework-for-the-nhs-in- england-2012-13 (Accessed 11 June 2014).

DH (DEPARTMENT OF HEALTH). (2012) *Caring for our future: Reforming care and support*. Policy Paper. London: DH. Available at: https://www.gov.uk/ government/publications/caring-for-our-future-reforming-care-and-support (Accessed 4 August 2014).

DH (DEPARTMENT OF HEALTH). (2014) *Five year forward view*. Available at: http://www.england.nhs.uk/wp-content/uploads/2014/10/5yfv-web.pdf (Accessed 25 November 2017).

ETZIONI, D. A., LIU, J. H., MAGGARD, M. D. & KO, C. Y. (2003) The ageing population and its impact on the surgery workforce. Feature. *Annals of Surgery*, vol. 238, no. 2, 170–177. Available at: http://www.ncbi.nlm.nih.gov/pmc/ articles/PMC1422682/pdf/2003080000003p170.pdf (Accessed 4 May 2009).

FRANCIS REPORT. (2013) *Report of the Mid Staffordshire NHS Foundation Trust Public Inquiry*. Executive summary. Available at: https://www.gov.uk/ government/uploads/system/uploads/attachment_data/file/279124/0947.pdf (Accessed 10 July 2015).

GLENDINNING, C., JONES, K., BAXTER, K., RABIEE, P., CURTIS, L., WILDE, A., ARKSEY, H. & FORDER, J. (2010) *Home care re-ablement services: Investigating the longer-term impacts (prospective longitudinal study)*. University of York Social Care Policy Research Unit. Available at: http://php.york.ac.uk/inst/spru/pubs/1882/ (Accessed 3 June 2014).

HEWITT, C., LANKSHEAR, A., KAZANJIAN, A., MAYNARD, A., SHELDON, T. & SMITH, K. (2005) *Healthservice workforce and health outcomes: A scoping study*. Report. London: National Co-ordinating Centre for NHS Service Delivery and Organisation. Available at: http://citeseerx.ist.psu.edu/viewdoc/download?doi=10.1.1.473.7999&rep=rep1&type=pdf (Accessed 25 November 2017)

HYDE, P., MCBRIDE, A., YOUNG, R. & WALSHE, K. (2005) Role redesign: New ways of working in the NHS. *Personnel Review*, vol. 34, no. 6, 697–712.

THE INDEPENDENT. (2015). A million elderly people lack basic social care as unprecedented funding cuts leave struggling NHS to pick up the pieces, *The Independent*, 11 April. Available at: http://www.independent.co.uk/life-style/health-and-families/health-news/a-million-elderly-people-lack-basic-social-care-as-unprecedented-funding-cuts-leave-struggling-nhs-10170302.html (Accessed 3 August 2015).

INSTITUTE OF PUBLIC CARE. (2012) *Help to live independently, self-care and domestic tasks*. Retrieved from the Projecting Older People Population Information System (POPPI). Available at: http://www.poppi.org.uk/index.php?pageNo=348&PHPSESSID=gib2h5gbi7qd8ssvl49ubkq8l7&sc=1&loc=8640&np=1 (Accessed 2 February 2013).

INSTITUTE OF PUBLIC CARE. (2014) *Provision of unpaid care*. Projecting Older People Population Information System. Available at: http://www.poppi.org.uk/index.php?pageNo=328&PHPSESSID=gib2h5gbi7qd8ssvl49ubkq8l7&sc=1&loc=8640&np=1 (Accessed 10 June 2015).

INSTITUTE OF PUBLIC CARE. (2016) *Support arrangements*. Projecting Older People Population Information System. Available at: http://www.poppi.org.uk/index.php?pageNo=328&PHPSESSID=gib2h5gbi7qd8ssvl49ubkq8l7&sc=1&loc=8640&np=1 (Accessed 25 November 2017).

KING'S FUND. (2014a) *A new settlement for health and social care: Final Report*. Commission on the Future of Health and Social Care in England. London: The King's Fund. Available at: https://www.kingsfund.org.uk/publications/new-settlement-health-and-social-care (Accessed 25 November 2017).

KING'S FUND. (2014b) *Making best use of the Better Care Fund: Spending to save?* Evidence Summary. London: The King's Fund. Available at: https://www.kingsfund.org.uk/sites/default/files/field/field_publication_file/making-best-use-of-the-better-care-fund-kingsfund-jan14.pdf (Accessed 25 November 2017).

KING'S FUND. (2015) *Workforce shortages endanger delivery of the NHS five-year forward view*. Available at: http://www.kingsfund.org.uk/press/press-releases/workforce-shortages-endanger-delivery-nhs-five-year-forward-view (Accessed 12 November 2015).

LEWIN, G. F., ALFONSO, H. S. & ALAN, J. J. (2013) Evidence for the long term cost effectiveness of home care reablement programs. *Clinical Interventions in Ageing*, vol. 8, 1273–1281. Available at: http://www.silverchain.org.au/assets/

GROUP/research/Lewin-2013-evidence-for-the-long-term-cost-effectivenss-of-home-care-reablement-programs.pdf (Accessed 9 January 2014).

LEWIN, G. & VANDERMEULEN, S. (2010) A non-randomised controlled trial of the Home Independence Program (HIP): An Australian restorative programme for older home-care clients. *Health & Social Care in the Community*, vol. 18, no. 1, 91–99.

LGA (Local Government Association) & ADASS (Association of Directors of Adult Social Services). (2014) *Adult social care funding: 2014* State of the Nation *report.* Available at: http://cdn.basw.co.uk/upload/basw_111407-2.pdf (Accessed 25 November 2017).

LIU, J. X., GORYAKIN, Y., MAEDA, A., BRUCKNER, T. & SCHEFFLER, R. (2016) Global health workforce labor market projections for 2030. *Human Resources for Health*, vol. 15, no. 11, 1. DOI: 10.1186/s12960-017-0187-2.

MACKEY, H. & NANCARROW, S. (2004) Report on the introduction and evaluation of an assistant practitioner in occupational therapy. *Australian Journal of Occupational Therapy*, vol. 52, no. 4, 293–301. DOI: 10.1111/j.1440-1630.2005.00531.x.

NAIC (National Audit of Intermediate Care). (2013) *National audit of intermediate care*. All reports since 2012. Audit report. NHS Benchmarking Network. Available at: https://www.nhsbenchmarking.nhs.uk/projects/naic (Accessed 2 December 2017).

NAIC (National Audit of Intermediate Care). (2015) *National Audit of Intermediate Care: Summary Report.* Available at: https://static1.squarespace.com/static/58d8d0ffe4fcb5ad94cde63e/t/58f08efae3df28353c5563f3/1492160300426/naic-report-2015.pdf (Accessed 2 December 2017).

NANCARROW, S. A. (2004) Improving intermediate care: Giving practitioners a 'voice.' *Journal of Integrated Care*, vol. 12, no. 1, 34–42.

NHS ENGLAND. (2013) *The NHS belongs to the people: A call for action.* Available at: https://www.england.nhs.uk/2013/07/call-to-action/ (Accessed 10 July 2015).

NHS ENGLAND. (2016) *NHS Pay Review Body.* Review for 2014–15: Written evidence from NHS England, September. Available at: https://www.england.nhs.uk/wp-content/uploads/2016/10/nhse-initial-evidnc-nhs-prb-2016.pdf (Accessed 2 December 2017).

NHS ENGLAND. (2014) *Five year forward view.* Available at: https://www.england.nhs.uk/wp-content/uploads/2014/10/5yfv-web.pdf (Accessed 12 February 2015).

NHS INFORMATION CENTRE. (2009) *NHS hospital and community health services. Non-medical staff in England 1998–2008.* NHS Information Centre Workforce and Facilities Team. Available at: https://digital.nhs.uk/media/18158/NHS-Staff-1998-2008-Non-medical-Detailed-results-tables-pdf-/Any/nhs-staf-non-medi-1998-2008-rep2 (Accessed 2 December 2017).

OCLOO, J. & MATTHEWS, R. (2016) From tokenism to empowerment: Progressing patient and public involvement in healthcare improvement. *BMJ Quality & Safety.* vol. 25, 626–632. DOI: 10.1136/bmjqs-2015-004839.

PETER, L. J. & HULL, R. (2009) *The Peter Principle: Why things always go wrong.* New York: HarperCollins.

PSSRU (Personal Social Services Research Unit). (2013) *Changes in the patterns of social care provision in England*: 2005/6 to 2012/13. Discussion Paper No. 2867. London: PSSRU. Available at: http://www.pssru.ac.uk/archive/pdf/dp2867.pdf (Accessed 10 July 2015).

RAMESH, R. (2010) *Patients hit as NHS cash crisis forces big cuts. The Guardian*, 2 March. Available at: https://www.theguardian.com/society/2010/mar/02/nhs-primary-healthcare-trusts-cuts (Accessed 2 December 2017).

REILLY, M. (1961) Occupational Therapy can be one of the great ideas of 20th century medicine. 1961 Eleanor Clarke Slagle Lecture. *The American Journal of Occupational Therapy*, vol. 14, 87–105.

RT UK Question More. (2015) *Outrage over online bids for elderly care home contracts*. Available at: https://www.youtube.com/watch?v=nNeI1jSu2t0 (Accessed 3 August 2015).

SCIE (Social Care Institute for Excellence). (2011) *Reablement: Emerging practice messages*. Available at: http://www.scie.org.uk/files/EmergingMessages.pdf (Accessed 11 June 2014).

SCIE (Social Care Institute for Excellence). (2013) *Co-production in social care: What it is and how to do it*. Adult services: SCIE Guide No. 51. Available at: http://www.scie.org.uk/publications/guides/guide51/files/guide51.pdf (Accessed 20 June 2014).

SHIELD, F., ENDERBY, P. & NANCARROW, S. (2006) Stakeholder views of the training needs of an interprofessional practitioner who works with older people. *Nurse Education Today*, vol. 26, 367–376.

STANMORE, E. & WATERMAN, H. (2007) Crossing professional and organizational boundaries: The implementation of generic rehabilitation assistants within three organizations in the northwest of England. *Disability and Rehabilitation*, vol. 29, no. 9, 751–759.

THURSZ, D., NUSBERG, C. & PRATHER, J. (eds) (1995) *Empowering older people*. London: Cassell.

WANLESS, D. (2002) *Securing our future health: Taking a long-term view*. Final Report. London: HM Treasury. Available at: http://www.hmtreasury.gov.uk/d/chap5.pdf (Accessed 20 March 2010).

WANLESS, D. (2004) *Securing good health for the whole population*. Final Report. London: HM Treasury. Available at: http://webarchive.nationalarchives.gov.uk/+/http:/www.hm-treasury.gov.uk/media/D/3/Wanless04_summary.pdf. (Accessed 20 March 2014).

WFOT (WORLD FEDERATION OF OCCUPATIONAL THERAPISTS). (2016) *About occupational therapy: Definition 'occupation'*. WFOT Available at: http://www.wfot.org/AboutUs/AboutOccupationalTherapy/DefinitionofOccupationalTherapy.aspx. (Accessed 12 January 2016).

WOODFORD, H. J. & GEORGE, J. (2010) Intermediate care for older people in the UK. *Clinical Medicine*, vol. 10, no. 2, 119–123.

2

The Centrality of 'Service Users' in Reablement

V. Ebrahimi and S. Phillips

Chapter outline

Reablement has the potential to be one of the main avenues in not only managing the costs of an ageing population, but as an initiative which truly embodies the concept of personalisation. Personalisation and person-centred planning is evident in a number of government drivers: in England in 2007 with the agenda Putting People First (DH 2010); the Better Health, Better Care: Action Plan in Scotland (NHS Scotland 2007); and in Wales as early as 1989 (Wilson 1992). Some professions, however, would argue that practising in a client or person-centred manner has always been a core value and a fundamental objective. Occupational therapy (OT) is one of those. Enabling, enhancing and empowering people towards better health and well-being, through purposeful and meaningful occupation, is the ultimate focus of OT. More recently, however, people with **long-term conditions** (LTC) report a lack of involvement in care planning (NHS England 2015), with many – despite wanting to be autonomous at home – saying that a lack of support and information prevents them from doing so (IPPR 2014). This is surprising, particularly considering the emphasis by the Department of Health for services as well as practitioners, and indeed all health and social care workers, to be people-centred. Given the choice, most older people would choose to continue living at home over a residential tenancy, nursing home or other assisted living facility. Personalisation and perspectives relating to control are therefore inextricably linked and should be apparent in the reablement process and during interactions right through to the end of service provision.

While recognising personalisation as an important element, this chapter's aim is to continue clarifying what occupation is and its associated meaning, but more importantly what people make of it. In addition, the principles of person-centredness are explored from the perspective of the professions responsible for the delivery of reablement, but, more importantly, what person-centred means to recipients. This chapter will enable you to recognise the association between occupational engagement and health as well as factors associated with ageing in this context. We know this is important because of the earlier discussion in Chapter 1 about reablement: the concept, the process and as a particular philosophy or way of being. Alongside networks of support and relevant policy, the chapter will conclude with collective perceptions of reablement and the movement towards co-production.

Chapter objectives

By the end of this chapter you should be able to:

➤ Determine in more depth what person-centredness is and its relationship with personalisation agendas

➤ Define occupation and occupational engagement

➤ Appraise the link between occupational engagement and health

➤ Recognise how society perceives ageing as well as those who have reached later adulthood

➤ Determine people's perceptions of occupation and the concept of reablement

➤ Identify how moving towards co-production is the way forward

Person-centred practice and the personalisation agenda

Before discussing how people understand and perceive occupation and reablement services, we need to return to the idea of person-centred practice and its association with the personalisation agenda. The following provides an overview from the professions involved in the delivery of reablement and includes a collection of definitions. This is then followed by a discussion on what people consider to be the characteristics which demonstrate person-centred practice.

The health care professions' perspective on person-centred practice

At the start of the twenty-first century the National Service Framework (DH 2001) described person-centred care as care that respects others as individuals and is organised around their needs. In a review of the changes that this guidance achieved, further action was identified five years later by the Commission for Healthcare Audit and Inspection (2006). A key area for action was defined as:

> A change in culture ... moving away from services being service led to being person centred, so that older people have a central role not only in designing their care with the combination and type of service that most suits them, but also in planning the range of services that are available to all older people.

(p. 9)

Reflection Point 2.1   The meaning of person-centred practice

In your practice, or as a student or support worker, think about what person-centred practice means to you. Make a list below of some words you would associate with this kind of working:

_____

_____

Let's take this further in an example from nursing whereby it is suggested that it is not possible to distinguish between good quality nursing care for older people, and 'person-centred care'. Some question if they are not actually the same thing (Morton 1999 quoted in McCormack 2004). Nolan and colleagues (2004) prefer the term 'relationship-centred care', arguing that the term person-centred does not take into account the context in which people live, and the roles of families, friends, neighbours and others. The core philosophy of nursing practice is, in the main, based on 'caring for' rather than the 'hands-off' approach typically seen in the OT profession and reablement. Of course in the instance of rehabilitation nurses we would argue otherwise. Some interesting conclusions were reached, however, in a **concept analysis** on patient participation. In a review (Sahisten et al. 2008) of some international nursing literature to determine what this might look like, the following characteristics repeatedly appeared:

➤ An established and connecting relationship

➤ Surrendering of some power or control

➤ Shared information and knowledge, and an active mutual engagement in intellectual and/or physical activities

While this study was carried out in Sweden, with a caution that concepts change over time, the ideas clearly resonate with those found in much of the available literature in the UK today. Another relevant debate occurred in the OT profession, and in others, in terms of what to call the individuals that require health-related and social care services. Consider the questions raised in Reflection Point 2.2.

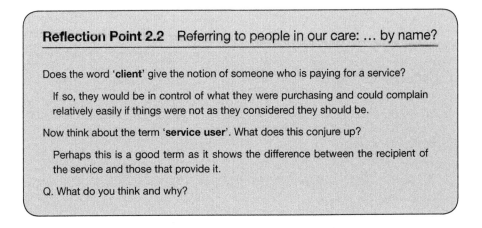

Reflection Point 2.2   Referring to people in our care: ... by name?

Does the word '**client**' give the notion of someone who is paying for a service?

   If so, they would be in control of what they were purchasing and could complain relatively easily if things were not as they considered they should be.

Now think about the term '**service user**'. What does this conjure up?

   Perhaps this is a good term as it shows the difference between the recipient of the service and those that provide it.

Q. What do you think and why?

Either way some people might suggest that service user is a good way of describing the person. Others may consider service user as derogatory, as one student once said: 'It sounds like you are using up all the resources ... depleting it ... it is negative.' What is evident, however, is that in any given interaction (with whatever term is used to describe them) 'the person' should be central in all interactions. It is their body, mind and personhood, their environment and well-being that we are essentially influencing as professionals, students in practice and support workers. Whether we agree with this assertion or not, what the literature makes clear is the complexity of 'person-centred care', bringing in explorations of themes such as knowing the person, the centrality of values, a shift in control and seeing beyond a person's immediate needs (McCormack 2004). We are also obliged to consider the ideas relating to person-centred working given the extensive legislation and guidance for both health and social care delivery since the advent of the personalisation agenda.

Professional codes of practice and philosophy

Person-centred practice is evident in the education and to varying degrees in the practice of many health care professionals and support staff. From an **occupational therapy** perspective this philosophy is evident in an early definition of client-centredness by Law, Baptiste and Mills (1995) which embraces the notion.

Box 2.1   Occupational therapy

Client-centredness involves:

respect for a partnership with people ... recognising the autonomy of the individuals, the need for client choice in making decisions about occupational needs ... [and that services] fit the context in which a client lives.

(Law, Baptiste and Mills 1995, p. 253)

Person-centred practice is apparent within **nursing** guidelines, although it is not explicitly stated in the professional code of conduct. The Royal College of Nursing developed eight principles to guide nurse leaders in further enhancing quality of care in nursing. This document was developed in collaboration with the Nursing and Midwifery Council, patient and service organisations as well as the Department of Health (RCN 2010). Principle D of the document outlines the provision of person-centred care.

Box 2.2   Principle of Nursing Practice D

Person-centred care:

emphasises the centrality of the patient to his or her care ... Such an approach requires a workplace culture where person-centred values are realised, reviewed and reflected on in relation to the experiences of both patients and staff.

(Manley 2011, p. 37)

The Code of Professional Values and Behaviour for **physiotherapists** makes much the same reference to a person-centred approach to practice: 'putting patients' and clients' needs to the fore' (Chartered Society of Physiotherapy 2011). For **social work** there is no such specific mention of client/person-centredness by the Health and Care Professions Council (HCPC), but there is in the 2012–2022 strategy for social work in Northern Ireland. In relation to intervention the strategy states that person-centred social work practice involves 'work-ing with people in need and supporting their right to autonomy and self-management of their lives and/or care' (Health, Social Services and Public Safety 2012, p. 40). Reference to person-centred principles fea-ture throughout the strategy. In addition, the term 'autonomy', which is referred to on a number of occasions, resonates with much of the discussion in this book. Collectively evident from all these statements is that the professional values outlined all veer to the same conclusion: *to promote what is best from the individual's perspective.*

The art of being person-centred

Consider what the average person thinks about how person-centred care is demonstrated. Common sense would suggest that if the first question in Box 2.3 were asked of a 'service user' then the response would be: 'well yes … of course care has to be about the person!'

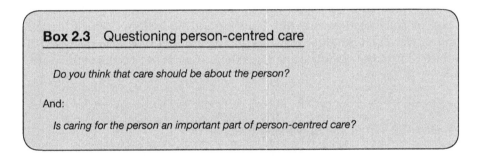

Box 2.3 Questioning person-centred care

Do you think that care should be about the person?

And:

Is caring for the person an important part of person-centred care?

Research carried out for the new nursing curriculum at the University of Manchester identified some strong themes. The research was conducted using focus groups of service users and carers, asking them about the qualities they sought in nurses (Griffiths et al. 2012). Overwhelmingly, the responses identified 'a caring professional attitude' as being a key quality. This was further articulated as 'empathy, communication skills, and non-judgemental patient centred care' (p. 121). One of the respondents com-mented that 'each individual should be assessed and their needs be assessed on that particular individual, rather than this is a basic rule for all', while another, an informal carer, stated: 'like getting to know you … you as a per-son what it is like for you and so that you don't have to explain all the time about yourself and the person you are caring for' (p. 124).

Here we see mention that the 'individual' is considered important. Recently, the Shaping Our Lives – National Network of Service Users and Disabled People was commissioned to review the standards of conduct, performance and ethics of the Health and Care Professions Council (HPC) (2014). The HPC comprises several professions and is a regulator whose aim is to protect the public. A focus group, which served as a consultation mechanism, with the participants being people who use services as well as their carers, indicated that compassion, empathy and reassurance were essential to the care continuum.

Box 2.4   Being clinical versus being human

In addition, the focus group for Shaping Our Lives – National Network of Service Users and Disabled People added:

> Sometimes personal conduct needs to be less medicalised and more human-ised. Meaning that when a disabled person comes into contact with any kind of practitioner there is a tendency to see disability [or problem or LTC] first and not the person.

(Shaping Our Lives 2013, p. 8)

See the person first, not the disability

The perspective outlined in this focus group is further reflected in a discussion on social care reform, supported by the Joseph Rowntree Foundation (JRF). This involved 27 people from a disparate and diverse range of adult social care services. While they welcomed the personalisation agenda, they viewed it at the time of the report as a process in which cuts to services were being justified, adding: 'to truly work, we need a cultural shift from social services staff' (JRF 2012, p. 19). This is extant in the discussion on the **ethos** of reablement throughout the chapters in this book in terms of cultivating a shift in thinking: how we view capability and potential in older community dwelling adults, and/or pre- or post-discharge from hospital settings. Although a small representative group nationally, inherently choice and control were not evident to these particular service users. The ideas of flexibility, choice and control, however, are echoed in government drivers in relation to the concept we know as personalisation.

Student Activity 2.1 Four principles for person-centred care and planning

Take a moment to examine the following four principles developed by a coalition of health and social care charities in 2013–2014 called National Voices. These are the processes, skills, behaviours and attitudes that were identified for person-centred care and support planning.

1. Prepare

➢ Starts from the point of view of the person

➢ Gathers necessary information and makes it available upfront

➢ Builds in time to reflect and consider options

2. Discuss

➢ Takes a partnership approach

➢ Focuses on staying well and living well (and, for some, it will also mean dying well)

➢ Identifies the actions that a person can take

➢ Identifies what care and/or support might be needed from others

3. Document

➢ The main points from discussions are written up, included as part of the person's health and/or social care records, and owned by the person and shared, with explicit consent

4. Review

➢ Considers options for follow-up and sets a date for review

Q. Do these processes, skills, behaviours and attitudes exemplify person-centred care and support planning?

Source: NHS England (2015, p. 13)

The parting message here is that all of these ideas, policies and guidelines are inconsequential. If the values we say we hold in relation to person-centred practice do not translate into subsequent behaviours, then we are deluding ourselves in a false **dichotomy**.

Personalisation

Personalisation has been driven by abundant **policy** initiatives. Indeed, in 1989, the Welsh Office published its 'Strategic Intent and Direction for the NHS in Wales', which identified person-centredness as central to its plans for health care (Wilson 1992). Instigated in 2007 in the UK, personalisation was introduced as a **radical reform** of social care which placed people at the forefront of services. The central premise of this agenda was for people to have more choice and control alongside early intervention and prevention (DH 2007). Today, the ideas are also intended to assist in aspects relevant to health care planning and more recently in **co-production**.

At a time of limited budgets, two seminars were held by the Social Care Institute for Excellence (SCIE) in 2012 to establish different per- spectives on personalisation. These seminars included people who use services, carers and those involved in policy and practice development in this specific area. When asked what personalisation meant to them in one of several workshops, one group produced a joint statement (SCIE 2012, p. 5):

➤ Personalisation for me is about: flexibility, choice and control

➤ To make it work for me, it needs peer support, information and advice

➤ If it's working well, it is liberating with positive outcomes

➤ I will be included and valued

➤ No decision about me, without me

➤ It's about being me

Other discussions reflected to a greater extent the above statements adding: 'the focus is on the person rather than the service – delivering quality of life and happiness and enabling you to live on your own terms' (SCIE 2012, p. 6). While there is no guarantee of enabling people to be happy, if quality of life (in terms of managing daily living) is even marginally perceived, then this is no doubt a move in the right direc- tion. In examining the language used and throughout chapters here so far, the link between person-centred care and personalisation becomes more apparent. Take a moment to look at Figure 2.1, which offers words associated with this approach to practice and working with people in your care.

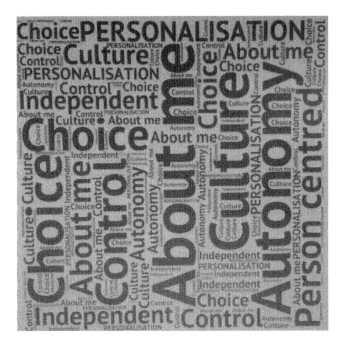

Figure 2.1   Inherent meaning in language and subsequent translations

Source: Created by Valerie Ebrahimi using Tagul online software (2015)

Student Activity 2.2   Inherent meaning in language and
subsequent translations: Negative connotations

List some phrases you have heard which mean the opposite to those presented in
Figure 2.1:

_____

_____

_____

_____

_____

Perhaps some of the phrases you came up with in Student Activity
2.2 included *'He is not compliant'* or *'She won't follow through with the*

care plan'. Maybe some of the ways in which we are not person-centred can be seen in our interactions, not our language. For example, a professional in uniform lowers their head and slumps their shoulders with an air of impatience when a person says that the prescribed equipment and intervention are not helping. A potential response and expression may be: 'Perhaps this is because you have recently been diagnosed with diabetes ... are you using it correctly?' – (not my fault) or worse (thinks 'non-compliant'). A better response might be: 'I am really glad you have told me about this. So ... rather than carry on struggling, let's see together whether another approach/aid will work. What do you think?' We can represent this more positive response in the following equation and then let's reflect further on language (see Reflection Point 2.3):

+ Communication   + Flexibility   + Partnership   + Individual Control
– Power versus Empowered +

Reflection Point 2.3 Personalisation

The word 'person' is at the beginning of **person**-alisation.

Let's assume that **'realisation'** is the final part.

Therefore, this may then lead us to ask another question:

Is person-centred care and support planning 'realised'?

Are the four principles identified by National Voices present in personalisation processes?

Today we have a number of services in health and social care aiming to demonstrate evidence of personalisation with varying degrees of success. Uniquely, reablement has the potential to achieve this and, it is argued, beyond, particularly from the perspective of a **paradigm** change in the way in which paid care is approached and provided from the outset. A paradigm change or shift is a movement from one way of thinking to another. Importantly for reablement this involves a renegotiation of the values of health and social care support staff and professionals as well as those that use services – a shift from 'doing to' to 'doing with' (Dewing 2004). Changes like this, however, do not happen quickly, but over time. We are unlikely to see this kind of change for another decade at least because often the move towards a radical culture shift is met with resistance in all corners of society. In an optimistic take on what the NHS might look like in 2030, by the charity Nesta (2015), one of the most fundamental changes, echoing the earlier equation, would be the interaction between people and professionals: '[a] shift [in] power towards the patient, creating more people-powered and person-centred care' (p. 23). It is not only a question of what this shift might look like and whether it would be evident across all services. It is a question of how NHS and social care services would instigate this, in light of their continued movement towards better and more effective integration.

Reablement – Understood

To a great extent reablement has the capacity to relieve some of the burden of care for family members, who also make up the collective body of people requiring services in their own right. One question that has yet remained unanswered, however, is whether those that use reablement services comprehend – in a broader sense of the term – what it is all about in the long term. Several studies and the literature in general indicate that people are often confused following hospital discharge as to what services they are receiving. A report in July 2015 found that very few patients felt they have been involved in their aftercare or in making decisions about it. The five main reasons cited (Healthwatch 2015, p. 10) for inadequate discharge include:

1. Experiencing delays and a lack of co-ordination between different services

2. Feeling left without the services and support needed after discharge

3. Feeling stigmatised and discriminated against and not treated with appropriate respect because of conditions and circumstances

4. Feeling a lack of involvement in decisions about care or given the information they need

5. Feeling that their full range of needs are not considered

Issues often arise during transitions from hospital to home and subsequent services, with recipients of reablement services often found to be confused. This was the case in the latter Scenario 1.2 with Barbara (see Chapter 1).

> *Who is involved in my care? Are you a nurse or an assistant? What is this reablement? Why are the [formal] carers not coming?*

Working on a joint project **The Pickering Institute** and the University of Oxford (2013) sought to fill in the gaps from the National Voices exercise – in other words, to better understand the key domains of integrated care and any information prioritising this initiative, but from the perspective of people who used the services. The overall aim was to improve on and develop new questions to measure people's experiences of integrated care. The outcome was to inform a limited set of questions to be included in seven national surveys. Among relevant evidence found, Cameron and colleagues (2014) reported that service users value certain indicators which might promote or hinder joint and integrated working between health and social care. These indicators were:

➤ Assessment, review and responsiveness to their needs

➤ Relationships and partnerships with named key workers

➤ Communication between agencies

➤ Information about complex systems

➤ Maintenance of independence

➤ Care planning

Penultimately, the 'I' statements in the overall review of evidence echoed much the same as that of National Voices: *my goals/outcomes; care planning; information; communication; decision making (including budgets); transitions (for example, a change from one service to another).*
Some statements matching the above 'I' statements included:

➤ *I want my GP to be the focus of my care*

➤ *I want my care to be better co-ordinated*

➤ *I want fewer repeat assessments*

➤ *I want my care to be local*

➤ *I want a person to be my key worker*

➤ *I want clear and easy-to-use information*

Some other reasons cited for inadequate discharge include stigmatisation and discrimination. This in itself is more disturbing and can be seen in examples such as Mid-Staffordshire (see the Francis Report 2013). Aside from person-centredness, explicit and foremost in all professional codes of conduct are the requirements to respect the people we work for and with, alongside equity of service provision and practices which are fair. This is an absolute and support staff, administrators, managers and ward clerks are equally bound to these principles.

A further complication in this **debate** is that recipients do not always comprehend fully what the aim or philosophy of reablement is. When this is the case the outcome may be disappointment at not being 'looked after'. This is particularly relevant in the instances where formal care has been in place for many years (Glendinning et al. 2010). Looking back at the statements in the Healthwatch (2015) report for inadequate discharge, number three – *'feeling left without the services and support needed'* – is clearly an issue. Yet, in order to establish more concrete evidence of this in relation to reablement services, further research is required. In addition, a clearer understanding is needed of what occupation means, not only to people who use reablement services, but also to their informal carers and the range of interdisciplinary professionals and support workers who deliver it. This is rightly so as it remains undisputed that:

> the vehicle for change in reablement is through occupation.

The value of occupation to health (body and mind) needs to be more explicit than it currently is, alongside the recognition that it has the potential to improve quality of life in older community-dwelling populations. Before considering the term occupation any further, it is necessary to understand how **social constructs** can negatively impact on change. This is because negative constructs will ultimately have a bearing on the paradigm shift mentioned in earlier discussions – from *'hands-on'* to *'hands-off'*.

The philosophy of reablement and occupation as a social construct

In its simplest terms, the philosophy of reablement can almost be described or considered as 'undoing a dependency'. In other words: to deconstruct and then rebuild (construct) an alternative paradigm (shift in thinking); to unravel existing ideas about how we live and how we demonstrate autonomy in later age. Dependencies are often created by the very services that seek to support people in times of need and these can often include **informal care** providers.

Reflection Point 2.4   More and more older carers are putting their health at risk

---

'The number of older carers in England is rising, with signs the pressures of look-ing after loved ones is damaging their health, research suggests. ...The warning by Age UK and Carers UK came as the charities released figures showing there were 1.2m carers over 65 – a 25% rise in the past decade.'

Q. What does the above suggest about the way our society considers ill health in older people?

Q. What about the role of the family and partners as carers?

Source: **BBC News, April 2015 (Triggle 2015)**

The idea of undoing dependency is a difficult paradigm or construct to embed, both at a practice level and for those older people who engage in reablement interventions, including families. Constructs are subjec-tive ideas and experiences about reality in everyday life. In simpler terms they define the meanings and notions that people have through everyday **social discourse** (dialogue) and interaction. 'Social' is added here because these ideas and realities can only be discovered through communicating with others or from our reading – whether implicitly (subconscious) or explicitly (conscious) these are embedded in our way of thinking. To undo what has been an integral part of people's expectations of health and social care services, that is paid care, is quite simply a monumental task. This will take time. In addition, a carer's paradigm, whether paid a sal-ary or not, is essentially one of 'doing for' rather than 'enabling to'. The expectation is that family and partners will do the caring and 'hands-on' tasks – that is until there is a significant breakdown in the ability to care. Reablement needs a balance between 'hands-on' (support) and 'hands-off' (facilitation). At the same time there is the need to recognise that some activities may simply need to be carried out for the person and that this is often okay. It is not okay, however, if this is to the detriment of family and partners, whether in later retired adulthood or still in employment. Of course the upshot of this is that although we may argue the value of being autonomous, we are nonetheless all interdependent at one time or another, whether or not we have a disability or a long term-condition. The question is whether or not we are getting the balance right.

Occupation: Different perspectives on the term

To demonstrate what a cultural shift in thinking might look like, we can take an example from the latter part of the 1960s – often associated as the true start of the **postmodern era**. Prior to this, much more of an emphasis on enhancing or 'fixing' component parts (of the individual) was evident in health services and subsequent interventions (Greber 2011). The focus at that time was on the malfunctioning limb – for example, a problem in mechanics in the upper right arm. It is a reductionist stance whereby, instead of considering other factors that impact on the person, the component part (the limb) bears more significance. This mode of thinking and practice is otherwise known as a structuralist approach (see Box 2.5). On the other hand, the pragmatist approach (inherently different) values 'holism': people are individuals (individualism) and other aspects are of equal importance, from their psychological health right through to the environment they live in. People therefore have their own personal stories to tell – their own truths about their condition, impairment or disability and the relationship of this to others in society. This is particularly important in our understanding of reablement, which is multifaceted, involving not just people who use these services, but others such as carers – both informal and formal. Formal paid carers are mentioned here because ultimately, they have a high level of face-to-face time with people and can often speak up for a person, although an **advocate**, in the absence of family, is often a better solution. The environment adds an equally important dimension here and the reason for this is more apparent in the discussions on assistive technology in Chapter 8. Pragmatist approaches add complexity to the whole equation, but ultimately can be argued as being far more person-centred than a structuralist one.

Box 2.5   A structuralist approach in practice

Martin had a cerebralvascular accident and as a result, the use of his right arm is limited.

This affects his range of movement (ROM) and he is unable to carry out PADL. The OT focus is on improving Martin's ROM by facilitating his ability to get dressed

▶

◀

independently. She does this, however without considering the social, emotive, familial and subsequent environmental issues.

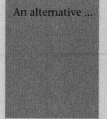

An alternative ...

... the pragmatist approach

By probing a little deeper, the OT discovers that Martin feels his impairment is very obvious to others when he goes out. To him this aspect is far more significant than his ability to manage his self-care.

The OT explores with him alternative ways of moving so that Martin can still be around others in a more relaxed way and therefore feel less socially isolated. They also explore together some inconspicuous aids for use in supermarkets, in the pub and so on, and, in an informal way, discuss the impact of the stroke on his masculinity.

Certainly there is a welcome change from structuralist to pragmatist approaches to practice today, which is clearly evident in the manner in which some reablement interventions are carried out. Goal setting is discussed in Chapters 3 and 5 alongside some of the challenges. To enable this approach, engagement between the professional or support worker and service user is essential in order to establish meaningful activities. There is not much point in working towards something that has little or no meaning to a person. Society's perceptions of 'ageing' are moving gradually from the idea of becoming dependent in later years to one of active ageing and **ageing in place**. Clearly this must involve people in defining and setting their own outcomes for interventions. Although these often focus around activities of daily living (PADL or DADL) (Lewin et al. 2013), which from a self-care context we readily identify with, activities such as walking the dog may be equally therapeutic, bringing forth a sense of, and connection with, local community or indeed society at large.

In Chapter 1 of this book we explored the meaning of the word 'occupation', defining it in broad terms as the activities or actions that a person or a number of individuals choose to engage in. Examples of these might include combing one's hair, stroking a cat, making a sandwich or going for a walk. These activities are not enforced, although there may be some societal pressure to carry out some of these, such as with personal activities of daily living (PADL). In the instance of PADL, it is reasonable to say that society generally has little tolerance for people who are malodorous (smelly). Being able to bath or shower is therefore quite important for those that are conscious of society's expectations (less so perhaps for the person with dementia). Suffice to say that all these, and other, activities involve tasks – smaller actions – that make up the whole. In the earlier example of tea making in Chapter 1, some of these tasks were described as involving **voluntary movement, positioning** and **cognitive processing**. In addition, occupation has intrinsic and extrinsic meaning. What is done (intrinsic – internal to self) has meaning to the individual and this then has an impact on others (extrinsic – external to self). Let's think about this using a common example (Scenario 2.1) from a practice situation.

Scenario 2.1   Amelia

Despite taking some time, Amelia and her experience of rheumatoid arthritis manages her self-care in the evenings following a reablement intervention. Amelia's husband gets to read his paper or watch the news as a result. As well as being able to do a leisure activity, his primary need for rest is also met. For Amelia, being able to wash her face, brush her teeth and undress has meaning to her in terms of autonomy and because it reduces the pressure on her husband to care for her. The couple also continue to be intimate. Helping a partner to wash, get dressed/undressed every day is more than likely to lower libido. Importantly, as Amelias is able to do this, her action also benefits her husband who is also a recipient of health and social care services (Care Act 2014).

Quite simply, in this scenario, by engaging in her own personal care, the occupation has dual influence. It has meaning from the point of view of autonomy, but also it enables others to take time out and enjoy occupations that have meaning to them.

Some more definitions of occupation

The term occupation has not changed that much historically. Definitions tend to draw towards the same initial conclusion: that occupation encompasses a person's job or profession, their usual or principal work and is a means to earn a living. Secondary to this, definitions involve the term 'activity', 'doing' or as the *Oxford English Dictionary* and *Collins English Dictionary* state: the action or act of occupying or the state of being occupied. When deconstructing (pulling apart) these two words, one of which is a verb (doing), it is evident, however, that two **phenomena** (observable experience), or as Immanuel Kant would argue noumenon (not directly accessible to observation), are at play. Although there are some criticisms of Kant's philosophy, within the context of this discussion, his ideas help to contextualise what is a somewhat complex state to grasp. This philosophy is explained in further detail in what follows and in relation to a common DADL: peeling potatoes.

Scenario 2.2   Peeling potatoes

Phenomenon – *'the action or act of occupying'* can be seen to a certain extent in a physical reality.

I can see you peeling potatoes.

Noumenon – *'the state of being occupied'* is an internal process which cannot be seen.

I cannot see what you are thinking but I know you probably are.

Understanding these two perspectives is important because during a reablement intervention there are two processes going on: one which is tangible and you can see; and the other which is private and sometimes withheld and not discussed.

What you can see – the person grasps the potato peeler in his left hand and starts peeling.

What you cannot see – the person deep in thought: *'Hmph ... Greta made my meals before she died. Wouldn't it just be easier to get someone to do this for me'* (frustrated and angry).

In Scenario 2.2 all seems well and the person is engaged in the activity, but it is a reluctant one. The question arises as to whether he would carry on with this activity once reablement services withdrew. It would be better to use the time more effectively – to engage with something that he wholeheartedly wants to achieve. Being able to capture or at least consider what is not directly observable is therefore important, as in this scenario. It is a basic principle of being person-centred. With more experience, visual cues that indicate anxiety can be observed – for example, shaking during an activity when this has not been present before and is not condition-related. Rubbing hands may indicate sweaty palms – a reaction from the **autonomic nervous system** (not controlled by conscious thought). The same can be said when a person responds to questions breathlessly, or if impatient or frustrated, the tone of voice and eye contact (or lack of) are observable. It is equally important, if not more so, to consider how people with an LTC might describe occupation. What it is and comprises of, to them, is often in stark contrast to the associated meaning for those who work in health and social care services. It is not possible to truly capture an individual's experience (noumenon), especially when ill health or an LTC is involved. At this point the statement in Harper Lee's story from the 1960s, *To Kill a Mockingbird*, has particular resonance:

> You never really understand a person until you consider things from his point of view ... until you climb inside of his skin and walk around in it.

(Lee 2010, p. 33)

The appropriate culture of compassion

It is valuable to hear people's explanations of what occupation is to them in the context of reablement services. This is necessary not only to gain an understanding of the personal meaning attributed to particular occupations, but also to create mutual understandings that a person is an expert of his or her own world, and the condition as it affects them. This, together with current trends for professionals to emphasise more compassion to those within their care, suggests a more **humanistic approach** to reablement. There is currently a lack of studies that explore how people perceive reablement or at least rehabilitation-specific services (Trappes-Lomax and Hawton 2012) and there are challenges to delivering a person-centred approach. We have only to consider the tensions created in a market-led service when referring to people as our 'clients' or 'service users' to note this is a depersonalised form of addressing people.[1] We must be mindful of the fact that although most of us would agree that health professionals should be compassionate, it is compassion that is frequently perceived as lacking and therefore lamented by patients, their families, policy makers, and health professionals alike (Smajdor 2013). A prime example is the public inquiry at the Mid Staffordshire NHS Foundation Trust (Francis Report 2013), where the key points led to evidence of an overarching negative culture in terms of:

➢ Professional disengagement

➢ Patients not being heard

---

[1] Acknowledgement to Michael Williams, Lecturer, University of Chester, for contribution on compassion.

➢ Poor governance

➢ Lack of focus on standards of service

➢ Inadequate risk assessment of staff reduction

➢ Nursing standards and performance

➢ Wrong priorities

As compassion is clearly valued we must guard against what Bradshaw (2009) describes as a McDonald's type of compassion where certain stocked behaviours and phrases are taken to embody its meaning. Further challenges to the 'personalisation of reablement' lie with the radical restructuring and financial pressures of health services, accused of reducing interpersonal care to task-focused routines, measured in terms of managerial agenda and staff shortages. Such health care failings prompted QC Francis in 2003 to propose that: 'There should be an increase on a culture of compassion and caring in nurse recruitment, training, and education' (Mid Staffordshire NHS Foundation Trust Inquiry 2013, p. 76).

When addressing reablement in the community, the Care Quality Commission (CQC 2014, p. 8) outlines five key questions of care professionals:

1. Are their clients *safe* in terms of protection from abuse and avoidable harm?

2. Is their client's care *effective* in terms of treatment and support to achieve quality of life based on the best available evidence?

3. Are they *caring,* in terms of treating clients with compassion, kindness, dignity and respect?

4. Are they *responsive* in terms of organising services to meet people's needs?

5. Are they well led in terms of management, learning and innovation to promote an open and fair culture?

Considering this, a compassionate person-centred approach to reablement is not only a requirement but also an expectation we must strive to live up to. Although the act of caring suggested by the CQC requires some degree of emotional investment on the part of the health care professional it proves surprisingly beneficial to them. Behavioural research suggests that when we engage in acts of soothing, calming and reassuring with others we also gain psychological reward due to the positive effects from oxytocin and opiate release to our emotional centre at such times

(Neff 2012). Therefore, when we take time to actively listen, to remain silent and not offer our opinion, we truly engage in partnership with people. This is often motivating, if not satisfying for both, as it enables a connection and perhaps mutual understanding which in turn fosters trust – argued here as an important aspect of a person's reablement journey. Indeed, this quality is identified in Griffiths and colleagues' (2012) research as being an essential quality in nurses.

Returning to the example of Greta's husband, observing in silence and then asking later on what a person's thoughts are about using a potato peeler, is an example of compassion and effective engagement. In this instance, by sitting back and not being afraid or wary of silence, the person involved in enabling allows the other to really engage and feel what it is like to carry out the task. Do we have to bring in our opinion at all? Can we let people be the judge of what the activity brings to them – whether it is purposeful or, better still, what meaning/s they associate with it? Jeremy, a person who has used health services extensively, offers an interesting perspective that relates to earlier discussions about the mind–body link. This example demonstrates only one opinion about what occupation is, but it is nevertheless rather astute.

Jeremy describing occupation:

> 'It is doing things to assist the well-being of your physical being and your mind ... to just occupying yourself.'
>
> **(Kindly provided by a Focus-NW group member)**

It is also interesting to see here the parallel between Reilly's (1961, p. 88) statement in Chapter 1 (Reflection Point 1.1) and the acknowledgement of Jeremy, that in the act of doing one 'is energized mind, body and soul'. On the other hand, the comment 'just occupying yourself' could resonate with something that has little if no meaning. Perhaps Scenario 2.2 with the potato peeling activity illustrates what will be discussed in Chapter 7 on disengagement theory: the gradual withdrawal from society and the reduction in strain and stress of leading a fuller life. At this point it is useful to take this idea further because it is here that the link between the ideas of control and health becomes more pervasive. First let us consider what some of the contemporary views on ageing are from the position of the UK as well as some international perspectives.

Shifting ideas about 'late old age'

Said the little boy, 'Sometimes I drop my spoon.'
Said the old man, 'I do that too.'
The little boy whispered, 'I wet my pants.'
'I do that too,' laughed the little old man.
Said the little boy, 'I often cry.'
The old man nodded, 'So do I.'
'But worst of all,' said the boy, 'it seems
Grown-ups don't pay attention to me.'
And he felt the warmth of a wrinkled old hand.
'I know what you mean,' said the little old man.

(Silverstein 1981, p. 95)

One of the most well-known definitions or conceptualisations of **successful ageing** was put forward in 1997 by Rowe and Khan. They proposed that there are three main constituents for this: '[a] low probability of disease and disease-related disability, high cognitive and physical functional capacity, and active engagement with life' (Rowe and Khan 1997, p. 433). They contended that successful ageing is more than absence of disease, however, and this reflects the earlier discussions about the structuralist/reductionist versus more pragmatic approaches to health provision. Furthermore, although functional capacity or capability is deemed important, Rowe and Khan assert that: 'it is their combination with active engagement with life that represents the concept of successful aging most fully' (p. 433).

The image that Silverstein's poem conjures is multifarious and, in light of the above definition on successful ageing, it is in stark contrast. On one end of the spectrum the old man is seen as childlike is relevant to **infantilism** and is described in more depth in Chapter 4. These childlike characteristics are defined in terms of incapacity – 'I drop my spoon ... I wet my pants ...' – but the striking message here is one of feeling undervalued and invisible, not part of mainstream society. From an equally ominous perspective, Phillipson (2013) refers to the pressures society has placed on our ageing population, with the emphasis that one should strive to be one of the 'well elderly'. This he described in terms of active and successful ageing – omnipresent in a range of literature. In the instance, for example, of the UGA Institute of Gerontology (2012), a whole website is devoted to this discussion (via social media) with a series of five published papers debating the concept.

Returning again to the poem, note too the language: 'the little old man' – ageist and oppressive in nature. Given popular culture and imagery often seen in adverts and birthday cards and so on, the traditional stereotypical image of the older person has been exacerbated by media representation, a portrayal of what youth is and what it should look like. The term 'fountain of youth' encapsulates how industry has profited on making a disease out of getting old. Despite being written in the context of the media in the USA, which has not been without some criticism there, clearly the issues Weintraub (2010) raises resonate in the UK. Steroids and 'anti-ageing treatments' such as Botox, have taken a bold leap forward from an industry that once only sold regenerating skin creams and make up, to that of 'smoothing wrinkles'. It is testament to the desire to avoid getting old, or at least looking older. Even women as young as eighteen are turning to cosmetic surgery, although this could be argued to some extent being related more on the ideal of having the 'perfect form', it nonetheless feeds into early insecurities about age and the ageing body. If a long-term condition, which invariably means that a person has a disability and/ or impairment, is added to this scenario, it is clear that ability or activity will also be measured in society according to age. These social constructs permeate at an individual level affecting among other things, self-concept as well as social relationships. The following statement demonstrates this issue. It was a comment made by a participant involved in a service evaluation: 'I've always been one that's been able to do for myself. But I'm not clever at talking to people. And now I've come to a complete stop' (Newton 2012, p. 120). Another more direct one made by a 75-year-old woman in relation to her difficulty using a computer: 'Well, we have to make way for the new and... out with the old [said dismissively with jovial laughter]' (personal communication 2013).

Other comments reflecting low self-concept were identified in a study (Connors, Kenrick and Bloc 2013) which sought to find out the views of older people using services in rural areas. Some of the thoughts expressed include the following:

> An attitude of 'making do' with what they have

> Not wanting to be a 'burden' on others

> Fear of admitting need and denial about the implications of ageing

> Low expectations of services and a feeling of personal responsibility

Newton (2012) argues, in relation to social rehabilitation, that person-centred approaches to reablement are based on the premise that 'what matters to the *individual*' (p. 119, emphasis added), in this case the older person, is what will promote their *individual* well-being. Arguably, in any context, if an activity has meaning to an individual they are going to want to engage with it and well-being may naturally follow. On the other hand, some occupations are detrimental to our health – for example, unhealthy food consumption and smoking. We may feel good when we finally get to light up that cigarette or eat that cake, but evidence points to a certain level of anxiety after the activity – or at least for most. Spending more time engaging in activities which make us happy requires active engagement. It means being truly present and in the moment. Much has been written in recent years about this mindset – in particular on the concept of mindfulness.

Moving minds to healthy places

The term mindfulness is not new, its philosophy spans thousands of years, although many have taken a great interest in its teachings since around 2013. Once considered a new-age concept, mindfulness involves refining awareness, or increasing attention, and is a flexible state of mind. Perhaps one of the first, or at least a pioneer of this, was Ellen Langer whose work has explored this concept in relation to older adults since the early 1960s. She consequently offers some very relevant perspectives on this idea that go hand in hand with the philosophy of reablement.

Langer (2010) discusses how we are all subject to psychopathologising everyday life. Rather than seeing sadness in some circumstances as rational, depression is the label given. Assumptions abound that a person who struggles to walk is going to avoid it for fear of falling. Anyone who has a difficulty with mobility must be depressed. These attitudes are very likely given the risk-aware society we live in. The question, however, is who is overly risk-averse here – 'service user' or professional? Once diagnosed, many service users build ideas about what will come next. In an age of technology, we are all guilty of self-diagnosing and searching for answers to our symptoms. These supposed certainties, however, harden our minds against possibility. This 'mindset' needs to be reversed in reablement interventions – putting our minds in a 'healthy place'. Mindfulness is simply about taking control of our thinking, to be aware of the present and be fully engaged rather than wondering what might come next.

One of Langer's (2010) studies demonstrates aptly how mindsets can be altered. In 1981 she took two separate groups of older men in their 70s and 80s to a monastery. The first group were left for a week and asked to pretend to be young men living in the 1950s. The environment was altered with magazines from that era alongside furniture from the mid-century, including a black and white television. The men discussed political events of that time, the need for bomb shelters (Cold War) and they heard the 1959 horse race commentary of Royal Orbit's win on a vintage radio. Had they been women they might have watched the opening of the Royal Ballet School by Princess Margaret in the same year and some would have enjoyed watching the film *Anatomy of a Murder* with Jimmy Stewart. The second group of men were asked to simply reminisce about the 1950s, and for this group lots of memories came to the forefront when they were asked about the horse race. Remarkably, however, the first group described the race as if it had taken place for the first time – as if they had only just participated in that 'glorious moment' of victory.

This is all well and good but it is quite reasonable then to ask what these examples and mindfulness have to do with shifting ideas about old age and reablement. The answer is relatively simple. In order to engage in activities of daily living with mindfulness, there is a need for people to move from what *might be* to *here I am in the moment* – to seize or take possession of the occupation. For us – as professionals, support staff, family and friends – there is a need to let go of the assumptions made for this age group about ability, capability and competence, or indeed, as many will testify, lowered expectations. Recall the phrase used earlier in Chapter 1: 'Competence … is in the eye of the beholder.' Let us now move on to explore the link between mindfulness, competence and meaningful occupations.

Meaningful occupation

> 'The Latin root word "occupatio" mean[s] to seize or possess.'
>
> (Yerxa et al. 1989)

In the mid-1980s there was a growing interest in understanding occupation (synonym 'doing') from a different perspective to that of the reductionist or structuralist era. Occupational science emerged in the late 1980s as a result of this, with its primary concern being with the form, function and meaning of occupations (Zemke and Clark 1996). Yerxa and colleagues (1989) explored the origin of the word occupation which is taken from the Latin root 'occupatio', meaning to seize or take possession. This is consequently a very important concept in relation to reablement.

Occupational science involves the study of human occupation – its nature and essence, and as Wilcock (1999) states: 'It is impossible to envisage the world of humans without it' (p. 1). In essence those that pro-vide reablement and those that receive it must recognise, and importantly accept, that humans are occupational beings. In relation to older peo-ple, two aspects that enable successful ageing might include meaningful occupational engagement and acceptance, as well as justice in the form of equal opportunity. This is argued, in the context of reablement and the earlier definition provided by Rowe and Khan (1997), as additional considerations for successful ageing. Reablement offers the older person with LTCs the opportunity to achieve personal goals that are relevant to them – meaningful engaging activities that are fulfilling in their everyday life. At this juncture it also provides the additional prospect for greater engagement with local communities. Active ageing from this perspective embodies occupational justice and, importantly, acceptance from others as capable, competent people with the ability to continue learning. But it also adds a social dimension that is most often lacking in health and social care intervention.

Occupational engagement and health

The idea that occupation can restore function is not new in con-temporary society (Molineux 2011). In 'doing' we 'act' and then 'become'. Acting and taking action is aptly described in Occupational Terminology (2005) as being 'linked to the development of abilities, skills and competencies, independence, identity, health and wellness' (p. 191). Research carried out through the years, and highlighted by Whalley-Hammel (2004), further demonstrates that making use of time through meaningful occupations 'restores a sense of value and purpose to life' (p. 300).

> 'When I am gardening nothing else matters ... lost is a good way to describe it. Well, I don't really feel conscious – you know what I mean? It kind of happens [acts out the movement] without thinking ... I mean pruning ... weeding that sort of thing.'

In the above quote, the individual is fully engaged in doing, and to some extent the activity of pruning and weeding seems therapeutic. Implicit in the words 'it kind of happens without thinking' is the suggestion of *being in the moment*. We can assume this from the woman's subsequent statement:

'I feel alive when I am in the garden pottering around, fiddling with the pots [thought-ful] … looking out for new growth. It makes me feel closer to Ben [her deceased hus-band]. I often find myself smiling at the bees … well, sometimes talking to them, but don't tell anyone [grins]'

Here the woman is 'becoming' and is enlivened by a meaningful activity. Identity might be closely linked to her feelings and thoughts for her deceased husband as a once married woman, but on the other hand not necessarily. This is clearly a very personal moment and we do not really need to know the what or why. It is simply an activity that works, needing no explanation.

There is another dimension to occupation and health which can be maladaptive, meaning that some occupations undertaken can harm people, in both a physical, psychological and cognitive capacity. A good example of this is during the **manic stage of bipolar** disorders or when skipping safety precautions when using ladders or lifting heavy items. Returning to Reflection Point 2.4 on carers putting themselves at risk of ill health, we can see the logic in this. Older carers engage in occupations of daily living for themselves, but they then add to this by seeing to the OATs of others. These tasks then become a burden. The person is over-occupied. This leads to the natural consequence of ill health, strain on relationships, a shift in control and more often little pleasure in daily living itself.

Research carried out prior to the turn of the twenty-first century investigated the risk factors specifically related to independent activities of daily living (IADL) and **mortality**. Ginsberg and colleagues (1999) found that those that were dependent on more than one instrumental activity of daily living (IADL) had a higher mortality risk. IADL is a term for activities that allow autonomy or independent living in the community such as shopping and looking after a pet. These activities are not associated with functional ones or primary needs such as personal care. Participants who had been bedridden two weeks, or more prior to the interviews, with cognitive impairment and had one IADL dysfunction, died over the six-year study. The researchers used logistic regression controls to take account of factors such as smoking and social status which may well have influenced the death rates, rather than IADL and health alone. A later study involving a random sample of 598 people over the age of 65 found that: 'there is a significant association between age, gender and dependence, as well as between dependence and morbidity and mortality, so that dependence could be used as a predictor of both' (Millán-Calenti et al. 2010, p. 306). Exploring these ideas further, and in their review of ADL-relevant literature, Mlinac & Feng (2016) found that the research evidence between 1998 and 2003 pointed to an increased risk of mortality and institutionalisation where individuals were dependent on ADL support. It could be argued then that despite today's surgical advances and ability to extend life, the issues relevant to dependence and perhaps quality of living remain a pertinent factor – they have not changed. The drive to do pleasurable tasks, not just those of necessity, remains a strong influencing factor in people's state of well-being. Will more research be carried out then to determine the benefit of leisurely and social activities? Can we already imagine the outcome?

A long-term study spanning the period 1993–2007 sought to establish the long-term decline in ADL, IADL and mobility among 5,871 older adults (Wolinsky et al. 2011). The method of the research was to link data from claims made through Medicaid (one of the most substantial insurance providers in the USA). The most significant finding was that frequency of hospitalisation and greater average annual number of admissions was the most robust indicator of functional decline. Perhaps the results of the study by Ginsberg and colleagues (1999) and Millán-Calenti and colleagues (2010) support preventative interventions such as reablement. What is certainly agreed, however, is that the longer people are kept out of hospital and encouraged to carry out meaningful ADL, the better. This latter comment takes us to the final concept discussed in this chapter.

Forwards to co-production

Although personalisation is relatively new to practice in the twenty-first century, it has been around for quite some time. The emergence of the Union of the Physically Impaired Against Segregation (UPIAS) (discussed in more depth in Chapter 4) in the 1970s is possibly the most evident early example of inching towards personalisation. This was during an era of collective movement towards co-production; people with disabilities took a stand against **institutionalisation**, asserting their right to live in the community. The concept of co-production is therefore not a new one. It seems to have been first coined in the 1970s when a professor offered an explanation of why crime rates went up when policemen returned to their patrol cars (NEF 2008). The suggestion here was that the police needed the community as much as the community needed them and that it was better to remain as much as possible 'on the beat'. Anna Cole, among others, used the term again at the Institute for Public Policy Research (IPPR), explaining that doctor–patient relationships fail when their need for each other is forgotten (NEF 2008).

For a paradigm shift, or ideas presented in reablement to take a hold in society, there needs to be a concerted movement across health and social care. We need the people who use our services to help us to succeed in this endeavour, but we also need their families and neighbours on board too. Envisaging the possibility of everybody coming together, pooling their resources, pooling their abilities and building on each other's potential, both to identify problems and then to solve them, would be one way forward. The words of Ruth Dineen, Director of Co-Production in Wales, resonate these ideas further when she describes the key features of co-production:

> [It's about working] together in equal and reciprocal relationships, so it is not the professionals coming in as experts and talking to citizens, and maybe consulting them about what's the best way of going forward, it's about citizens and professionals absolutely working together and understanding that both share power and both share responsibility.
>
> (Dineen 2014)

Work ongoing in Liverpool may be testament to co-production and this is discussed in more detail in Chapter 4. This will not be the case, however, if the ideas and thoughts of the community are not truly taken into account.

If we work in three different camps – the NHS, Social Services AND the public – what do we hope to achieve?

Law, Baptiste and Mills' (1995) early perspective on client-centredness hints at co-production as 'the involvement of service users', which although, as SCIE (2013) argues, has no singular formula, offers a number of definitions, to include the following shared definition:

> A relationship where professionals and citizens share power to plan and deliver support together, recognising that both have vital contributions to make in order to improve quality of life for people and communities.
>
> (National Co-Production Critical Friends 2013)

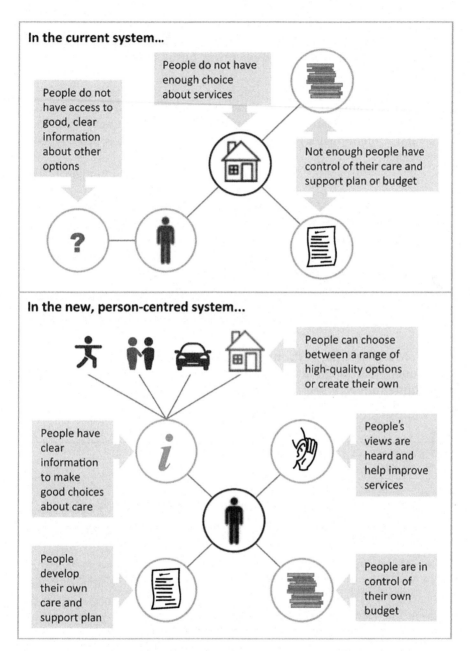

Figure 2.2   What will the future look like …? The vision for care and support detailed in the White Paper *Caring for our future: Reforming care and support*

Source: DH (2012, p. 9)

From a policy perspective, and as early as 2004, Stephen Ladyman, former Parliamentary Under Secretary of State for the Community, described not only the value of person-centred planning, but implicitly a move towards co-production:

> By 'person-centred' I mean we have to move away from mass produced services – services that too often created a culture of dependency – and move towards a future that seeks to develop the potential that is in every single individual.
>
> (Ladyman 2004)

What is this potential? How can we achieve it and how can reablement help in the movement towards this ideal? The strong link to personalisation is evident in co-production. SCIE (2013) describes it as a culture of equality where everyone has assets – a move away from problems and (the traditional) unequal relationships between service user and professional (and of course support worker). Here the link between the discussion in Chapter 4 on dominant ideologies and service land comes to the fore. This is well worth reading to make sense of what has been discussed so far.

We will continue with further discussion and deliberation about co-production throughout this book; however, the message it brings is really quite simply: *people are 'our economy'.*

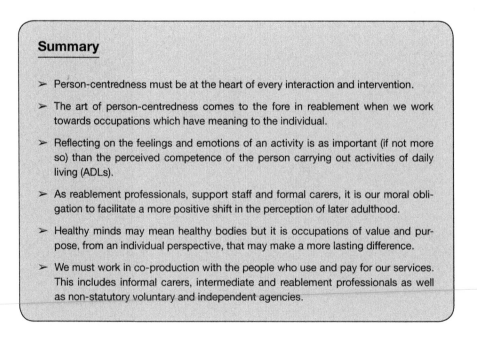

Summary

➤ Person-centredness must be at the heart of every interaction and intervention.

➤ The art of person-centredness comes to the fore in reablement when we work towards occupations which have meaning to the individual.

➤ Reflecting on the feelings and emotions of an activity is as important (if not more so) than the perceived competence of the person carrying out activities of daily living (ADLs).

➤ As reablement professionals, support staff and formal carers, it is our moral obligation to facilitate a more positive shift in the perception of later adulthood.

➤ Healthy minds may mean healthy bodies but it is occupations of value and purpose, from an individual perspective, that may make a more lasting difference.

➤ We must work in co-production with the people who use and pay for our services. This includes informal carers, intermediate and reablement professionals as well as non-statutory voluntary and independent agencies.

Recommended reading

HAMMEL, K. W. (2006) *Perspectives on disability and rehabilitation: Contesting assumptions; challenging practice.* Edinburgh: Churchill Livingstone.

IPPR (INSTITUTE FOR PUBLIC POLICY RESEARCH). (2014) Patients in control: Why people with long-term conditions must be empowered. Available at: www.ippr.org/assets/media/publications/pdf/patients-in-control_Sept2014.pdf

NHS ENGLAND. (2015) Personalised care and support planning handbook: The journey to person–centred care. Available from: http://www.england.nhs.uk/wp-content/uploads/2015/01/pers-care-guid-core-guid.pdf

For a more in-depth discussion on relevant policy see:

DOWLING, S., MANTHORPE, J., & COWLEY, S. (2006) *An exploration of the relevance of person-centred planning in social care.* Scoping Review. York: Joseph Rowntree Foundation, p. 12.

References

BRADSHAW, A. (2009) Measuring nursing care and compassion: The McDonaldised nurse? *Journal of Medical Ethics*, vol. 35, no. 8, 465–468.

CAMERON, A., LART, R., BOSTOCK, L. & COOMBER, C. (2014) Factors that promote and hinder joint and integrated working between health and social care services: A review of research literature. *Health and Social Care in the Community*, vol. 22, no. 3, 225–233. Available at: http://www.pickereurope.org/wp-content/uploads/2014/10/Developing-measures-of-IC-report_final_SMALL.pdf (Accessed 23 April 2015).

CARE ACT. (2014) *Care Act 2014: Part 1: factsheets.* Care Act Factsheet, HRMS. Available at: https://www.gov.uk/government/publications/care-act-2014-part-1-factsheets (Accessed 3 February 2015).

CHARTERED SOCIETY OF PHYSIOTHERAPY. (2011) *Code of members and professional values and behaviour.* Available at: http://www.csp.org.uk/publications/code-members-professional-values-behaviour (Accessed 3 January 2013).

COMMISSION FOR HEALTHCARE AUDIT AND INSPECTION. (2006) Living well in later life: A review of progress against the National Service Framework for Older People. Available at: http://www.scie.org.uk/publications/guides/guide15/files/livingwellinlaterlife-fullreport.pdf?res=true (Accessed 3 August 2015).

CONNORS, C., KENRICK, M. & BLOC, A. (2013) *Impact of an ageing population on service design and delivery in rural areas.* London: TNS BMRB and International Longevity Centre (on behalf of Defra). Available at: http://randd.defra.gov.uk/Default.aspx?Menu=MenuandModule=MoreandLocation=NoneandCompleted=0andProjectID=18501 (Accessed 10 January 2014).

CQC (CARE QUALITY COMMISSION). (2014) *The five key questions we ask.* Available at: http://www.cqc.org.uk/content/five-key-questions-we-ask (Accessed 12 December 2014).

DINEEN, R. (2014). *What is co-production?* 1000 Lives Improvement. YouTube video of Ruth Dineen, Director of Co-Production in Wales, speaking at the 1000 Lives Improvement Conference. Available at: https://www.youtube.com/watch?v=bo4r1XU-BZw (Accessed 12 January 2015).

DEWING, J. (2004) Concerns relating to the application of frameworks to promote person centredness in nursing with older people. *Journal of Clinical Nursing*, vol. 13, no. 1, 39–44.

DH (DEPARTMENT OF HEALTH). (2001) *The National Service Framework for older people*. Available at: https://www.gov.uk/government/uploads/system/uploads/attachment_data/file/198033/National_Service_Framework_for_Older_People.pdf (Accessed 2 June 2013).

DH (DEPARTMENT OF HEALTH). (2007) *Putting people first: A shared vision and commitment to the transformation of adult social care*. London: The Stationery Office. Available at: http://webarchive.nationalarchives.gov.uk/20130107105354/http:/www.dh.gov.uk/prod_consum_dh/groups/dh_digitalassets/@dh/@en/documents/digitalasset/dh_081119.pdf (Accessed 3 June 2013).

DH (DEPARTMENT OF HEALTH). (2010) *A vision for adult social care: Capable communities and active citizens*. Social Care Policy. Available at: http://webarchive.nationalarchives.gov.uk/20121107104731/http://www.dh.gov.uk/prod_consum_dh/groups/dh_digitalassets/@dh/@en/@ps/documents/digitalasset/dh_121971.pdf (Accessed 12 December 2017).

DH (DEPARTMENT OF HEALTH). (2012) *Caring for our future: Reforming care and support*. White Paper. Available at: https://www.gov.uk/government/publications/caring-for-our-future-reforming-care-and-support (Accessed 15 November 2014).

FLYNN, M. & MERCER, D. (2013). Is compassion possible in a market-led NHS? *Nursing Times*, vol. 109, no. 7, 12–14.

FRANCIS REPORT. (2013) Report of the Mid Staffordshire NHS Foundation Trust Public Inquiry. Executive summary. Available at: https://www.gov.uk/government/uploads/system/uploads/attachment_data/file/279124/0947.pdf (Accessed 10 July 2015).

GINSBERG, G. M., HAMMERMAN-ROZENBERG, R., COHEN, A. & STESSMAN, J. (1999) Independence in instrumental activities of daily living and its effect on mortality. *Aging (Milano)*, vol. 11, no. 3, 161–168. Available at: http://www.ncbi.nlm.nih.gov/pubmed/10476311 (Accessed 13 September 2014).

GLENDINNING, C., CLARKE, S., HARE, P., KOTCHETKOVA, I., MADDISON, J. & NEWBRONNER, L. (2006) *Outcomes-focused services for older people*. London: SCIE.

GLENDINNING, C., JONES, K., BAXTER, K., RABIEE, P., CURTIS, L., WILDE, A., ARKSEY, H. & FORDER, J. (2010) *Home Care Re-ablement Services: Investigating the longer-term impacts (prospective longitudinal study)*. York: University of York Social Care Policy Research Unit. Available at: http://php.york.ac.uk/inst/spru/pubs/1882/ (Accessed 20 June 2013).

GREBER, C. (2011) Pluralism: Signposting a split in occupational therapy? *Australian Occupational Therapy Journal*, vol. 58, 455–457.

GRIFFITHS, J., SPEED, S., HORNE, M. & KEELEY, P. (2012) A caring professional attitude: What service users and carers seek in graduate nurses and the challenge for educators. *Nurse Education Today*, vol. 32, 121–127.

HEALTHWATCH. (2015) *Safely Home: What happens when people leave hospital and care settings?* Available at: http://www.healthwatch.co.uk/sites/healthwatch.co.uk/files/safely_home_large_print_03082015.pdf. (Accessed 20 July 2015).

HEALTH, SOCIAL SERVICES AND PUBLIC SAFETY. (2012) *Improving and safeguarding social wellbeing. A strategy for social work in Northern Ireland. 2012–2022.* Available at: https://niscc.info/storage/resources/2012april_dhssps_socialworkstrategy2012-2022_afmck1.pdf (Accessed 10 December 2017).

HPC (HEALTH & CARE PROFESSIONS COUNCIL). (2014) *Review of the standards of conduct, performance and ethics. Thematic review: Collaborative approaches to care.* Available at: http://www.hpc-uk.org/assets/documents/1000463Eenc05-ProfessionalLiaisonGroupworkplan.pdf. (Accessed 3 February 2015).

IPPR (INSTITUTE FOR PUBLIC POLICY RESEARCH). (2014) *Patients in control: Why people with long-term conditions must be empowered.* Available at: www.ippr.org/assets/media/publications/pdf/patients-in-control_Sept2014.pdf (Accessed 24 June 2015).

Dowling, S., Manthorpe, J., and Cowley, S in association with King, S., Raymond, V., Perez, W and Weinstein, P.

JRF (JOSEPH ROWNTREE FOUNDATION). (2006) *Person-centred planning in social care.* York: JRF. pp. 1–64. Available at: http://www.jrf.org.uk/system/files/9781859354803.pdf (Accessed 20 June 2014).

JRF (JOSEPH ROWNTREE FOUNDATION). (2012) *Caring for our future: What service users say.* Brunel University and Shaping Lives. York: JRF. Available at: http://www.shapingourlives.org.uk/documents/caring-for-our-future-peter-beresford.pdf. (Accessed 2 February 2015).

LADYMAN, S. (2004) *Health and social care advisory service: New directions in Direct Payments for people who use mental health services.* Speech, Department of Health, London, 18 May. Available at: http://webarchive.national-archives.gov.uk/+/www.dh.gov.uk/en/MediaCentre/Speeches/Speecheslist/DH_4083721 (Accessed 2 February 2014).

LANGER, E. J. (2010). *Counterclockwise: Mindful health and the power of possibility.* London: Hodder & Stoughton.

LAW, M., BAPTISTE, S. & MILLS, J. (1995) Client-centred practice: What does it mean and does it make a difference? *Canadian Journal of Occupational Therapy*, vol. 62, no. 5, 250–270.

LEE, H. (2010) *To Kill a Mockingbird* (50th Anniversary edn). London: Arrow Books.

LEWIN, G., DE SAN MIGUEL, K., KNUIMAN, M., ALAN, J., BOLDY, D., HENDRIE D. & VANDERMEULEN, S. (2013) A randomised controlled trial of the Home Independence Program, an Australian restorative home-care programme for older adults. *Health and Social Care in the Community*, vol. 21, no. 1, 69–78.

MANLEY, K., HILLS, V. & MARRIOT, S. (2011) Person-centred care: Principle of nursing practice D. *Nursing Standard*, vol. 25, no. 31. Available at: https://www.rcn.org.uk/__data/assets/pdf_file/0004/377365/Nursing_Standard_Principle_D_April11_560KB.pdf (Accessed 10 February 2015).

MCCORMACK, B. (2004) Person-centredness in gerontological nursing: A review of the literature. *Journal of Clinical Nursing*, vol. 13, no. 3a, 31–38.

MID STAFFORDSHIRE NHS TRUST PUBLIC INQUIRY. (2013) *Executive Summary.* Inquiry chaired by Robert Francis QC. 1.185, p.76. London: The Stationery Office.

MILLÀN-CALENTI, J.C, TUBIO, J., PITA-FERNANDEZ, S., GONZALEZ-ABRALDES, I., LORENZO, T., FERNANDEZ-ARRUTY, T. & MASEDA, A. (2010). Prevalence of functional disability in activities of daily living (ADL), instrumental activities of daily living (IADL) and associated factors, as predictors of morbidity and mortality. *Archives of Gerontology and Geriatrics*, vol. 50, 306–310. Available at: http://www.ncbi.nlm.nih.gov/pubmed/19520442 (Accessed 14 September 2014).

MLINAC, M. E., & FENG M. C. (2016) Assessment of activities of daily living, self-care, and independence. *Archives of Clinical Neuropsychology*, vol. 31, no. 6, 506–516. Available at: https://doi.org/10.1093/arclin/acw049 (Accessed 12 December 2017).

MOLINEUX, M. (2011) Standing firm on shifting sands. *New Zealand Journal of Occupational Therapy*, vol. 58, no. 1, 21–28.

NATIONAL CO-PRODUCTION CRITICAL FRIENDS. (2013) *National Co-production Critical Friends' shared definition: Co-production.* Available at: http://api.ning.com/files/A1Qs8*3Ts4xAGEMdfQiEa21YSR8xlBKfFawmG5tQcDpcf2gBlmHBfL82ChkhblrDHzf3juE9cRk5LCFrxMfaM3LYxgOh4uUv/Shareddefinition.pdf (Accessed 6 May 2014).

NEF (NEW ECONOMICS FOUNDATION). (2008) *Co-production: A manifesto for growing the core economy.* Available at: http://b.3cdn.net/nefoundation/5abec531b2a775dc8d_qjm6bqzpt.pdf (Accessed 12 January 2014).

NEFF, K. (2012) *The physiology of self-compassion.* Available at: http://self-compassion.org/the-physiology-of-self-compassion/ (Accessed 13 February 2014).

NESTA. (2015) *The NHS in 2030: A vision of a people-powered, knowledge-powered health system.* Available at: http://www.nesta.org.uk/publications/nhs-2030-people-powered-and-knowledge-powered-health-system (Accessed 15 July 2015).

NEWTON, C. (2012) Personalising reablement: Inserting the missing link. *Working with Older People*, vol. 16, no. 3, 117–121. DOI: 10.1108/13663661211260934.

NHS ENGLAND. (2015) *Personalised care and support planning handbook: The journey to person–centred care.* Available at: http://www.england.nhs.uk/wp-content/uploads/2015/01/pers-care-guid-core-guid.pdf (Accessed 24 June 2015).

NHS SCOTLAND. (2007) *Better health, better care: Action plan.* Edinburgh: The Scottish Government. Available at: http://www.gov.scot/Resource/Doc/206458/0054871.pdf (Accessed 14 September 2014).

NOLAN, M. R., DAVIES, S., BROWN, J., KEADY, J. & NOLAN, J. (2004) Beyond 'person-centred' care: A new vision for gerontological nursing. *International*

Journal of Older People Nursing in association with Journal of Clinical Nursing, vol. 13, no. 3a, 45–53.

OCCUPATIONAL TERMINOLOGY. (2005) *Journal of Occupational Science,* vol. 12, no. 3, 191–194. DOI: 10.1080/14427591.2005.9686564.

PHILLIPSON, C. P. (2013) *Ageing: Key concepts.* Cambridge: Polity Press.

THE PICKERING INSTITUTE & THE UNIVERSITY OF OXFORD. (2013) *Developing measures of people's self-reported experiences of integrated care.* Available at: http://www.pickereurope.org/wp-content/uploads/2014/10/Developing-measures-of-IC-report_final_SMALL.pdf (Accessed 4 June 2014).

RCN (ROYAL COLLEGE OF NURSING). (2010) *Principles of nursing practice: Principles and measures consultation.* Summary report for nurse leaders. Available at: http://www.rcn.org.uk/__data/assets/pdf_file/0007/349549/003875.pdf (Accessed 21 February 2014).

REILLY, M. (1961) Occupational Therapy Can Be One of the Great Ideas of 20th Century Medicine. *The American Journal of Occupational Therapy,* vol. 14, no. 88, 87–105.

ROWE, J. W. & KAHN, R. L. (1997). Successful aging. *The Gerontologist,* vol. 37, no. 4, 433–440. DOI:10.1093/ geront/gnu074.

SAHISTEN, M. J., LARSSON, I. E., SJOESTROEM, B. & PLOS, K. A. B. (2008) An analysis of patient participation. *Nursing Forum,* vol. 43, no. 1, 2–11.

SCIE (SOCIAL CARE INSTITUTE FOR EXCELLENCE). (2012) *People not processes: The future of personalization and independent living.* Workforce development: Report No. 55. Available at: http://www.scie.org.uk/publications/reports/report55/ (Accessed 3 February 2015).

SCIE (SOCIAL CARE INSTITUTE FOR EXCELLENCE). (2013) Co-production in social care: What is co-production – Defining co-production. *Recommendations.* Available at: http://www.scie.org.uk/publications/guides/guide51/recommendations.asp (Accessed 12 December 2013).

SHAPING OUR LIVES. (2013) *Service User and Carer Consultation Review of the Standards of conduct, performance and ethics of the Health and Care Professions Council.* The National Network of Service Users and Disabled People. Available at: http://www.shapingourlives.org.uk/ourpubs.html#HCPC (Accessed 2 February 2015).

SILVERSTEIN, S. (1981) *A light in the attic.* New York: Harper Collins.

SMAJDOR, A. (2013). Reification and compassion in medicine: A tale of two systems. *Clinical Ethics,* vol. 8, no. 4, 111–119.

TRAPPES-LOMAX, T. & HAWTON, A. (2012) The user voice: Older people's experiences of reablement and rehabilitation. *Journal of Integrated Care,* vol. 20, no. 3, 181–194.

TRIGGLE, N. (2015) More older carers 'risking health'. *BBC News,* 30 April. Available at: http://www.bbc.co.uk/news/health-32520410 (Accessed 20 July 2016).

UGA INSTITUTE OF GERONTOLOGY. (2012) Healthy and successful aging project. Available at: https://healthyandsuccessfulaging.wordpress.com/author/jayneclamp/ (Accessed 20 June 2014).

WEINTRAUB, A. (2010) *Selling the fountain of youth: How the anti-aging industry made a disease out of getting old – and made billions.* Philadelphia, PA: Basic Books.

WHALLEY-HAMMEL, K. (2004) Dimensions of meaning in the occupations of daily life. *Canadian Journal of Occupational Therapy*, vol. 71, no. 5, 296–305. Available at: https://caot.ca/CJOT_pdfs/CJOT71/Hammell71%285%29296_305.pdf (Accessed 3 February 2015).

WILCOCK, A. A. (1999) Reflections on doing, being and becoming. *Australian Occupational Therapy Journal*, vol. 46, no. 1, 1–11.

WILSON, B. (1992) Establishing a people-centered health service in Gwent, Wales. *Journal of Healthcare Quality*, vol. 14, no. 3, 32–35. Available at: http://www.ncbi.nlm.nih.gov/pubmed/10119895 (Accessed 15 February 2015).

WOLINSKY, F. D., BENTLER, S. E., HOCKENBERRY, J., JONES, M. P., OBRIZAN, M., WEIGEL, P. A. M., KASKIE, B. & WALLACE, R. B. (2011) Long-term declines in ADLs, IADLs, and mobility among older Medicare beneficiaries. *BMC Geriatrics*. vol. 11, no. 43, 11–43.

YERXA, E. J., CLARK, F., FRANK, G., JACKSON, J., PARHAM, D., PIERCE, D. & ZEMKE, R. (1989) An introduction to occupational science: A foundation for occupational therapy in the 21st century. *Occupational Therapy in Health Care*, vol. 6, no. 4, 1–17.

ZEMKE, R. & CLARK, F. A. (1996) *Occupational science: The evolving discipline.* Philadelphia, PA: F. A. Davis.

3

Reablement Models of Service Provision

J. Greenwood, V. Ebrahimi and A. Keeler

Chapter outline

This chapter provides an introduction to the background of reablement services and guides the reader towards an understanding of the different methods of delivering reablement services. It considers some of the issues and challenges in provision of reablement and offers an insight into the future of these services in the UK.

Chapter objectives

By the end of this chapter you should be able to:

➤ Outline the historical development of reablement

➤ Provide an overview of different models of reablement within the UK

➤ Appraise the benefits and limitations of these models and approaches

➤ Consider the possible future developments in reablement

It is widely accepted across health and social care that the impact of and exponential increase in the older population has meant that the levels and design of services cannot remain the same (DH 2007b; Think Local Act Personal 2011; DH 2014a). Budgetary restrictions therefore continue to be a critical consideration in the planning of services. The result of this has meant dramatic changes in the way in which adult social care services are provided and will be provided in the future. Since their introduction, there appears to be no common agreement on the best way of providing reablement services. This has resulted in a myriad of approaches being adopted around the country (NEIEP 2010).

The approach to reablement – how the intervention is carried out and the process – is guided to a greater extent by a model. This is made up of theoretical and, in this instance, organisational knowledge, as well as innate or tacit knowledge learned from experience. This is then embedded in practice. There is no singular model of reablement. Some authorities have created reablement services from existing provision while others have developed new services. This might comprise care specific provision (domiciliary or care at home) or, as has often been the case until now, been delivered via occupational therapy (OT) services. In acute settings, such as hospitals, reablement can be found linked to rapid response services (attached to A&E and GP surgeries) or at the other end of the spectrum, community services linked to intermediate care or rehabilitation.

Successful reablement services are outcome-focused with the express aim of improving the health and well-being of the people that need them. Reablement seems to be more commonly associated in social care settings with or without joint funding from health care providers. Commissioners of adult social care are very aware of the evidence supporting the use of reablement services, not only for the short-term success in reducing budgets, but also for the longer-term benefits for the people that use them. In addition, these commissioners are having to think differently about how they provide services in order to keep within budgetary constraints. For instance, investing in a more preventative early intervention service, delaying the point at which people reach a crisis, negates extensive and costly social care schemes (McGregor 2013). The term care scheme is adopted over that of 'care packages' (commonly used in practice) as this language, however unintentional, depersonalises people. It moves away from notions of person-centredness, which is one of the key aims of this book.

Background and contemporary history of reablement

Reablement is defined in several different ways. It is often seen as an alternative approach to traditional home care, usually, although not exclusively, provided by social services departments within local authorities. Reablement was introduced with the aim of assessing and ideally minimising the need for ongoing long-term formal care. Supporting individuals to accommodate their illness or condition while learning or relearning the skills they need to live autonomously – is the key objective. Reablement, while sharing some features of other services, is distinguished by its impact on home care, veering away from the traditional care service model. In the words of Wood and Salter (2012):

The aim of reablement is not to do things for people, or to provide assistance, as in traditional homecare, but to show people how they can do things for themselves. Reablement workers may deliberately 'stand back' and offer encouragement without actively assisting people in carrying out daily tasks.

(p. 21)

Restorative care, as it is known in Australia, New Zealand and America, is described by Regan, Wells and Foreman (2009) as a movement away from a culture of dependency and co-dependency between carers, people using services and statutory services, to adopting a more 'can do' approach. This approach encourages people to maximise their independence or autonomy by offering frequent regular visits, which are usually time-limited in the UK to a maximum of six weeks (Cochrane et al. 2013) and during which time the person is not charged. Reablement in the UK has prompted a similar paradigm shift to that of Australia and the USA.

Meta-analysis of available evidence by Cochrane and colleagues (2013) sought to assess differences in usual paid care compared with reablement across the UK, Australia and USA, as well as costs/cost-effectiveness of reablement compared to conventional home care. The objectives were to assess whether there is a difference in functional independence in older adults who have received reablement interventions from a maintenance and improvement perspective. The results of this were yet to be published during the writing of this book. The first author, Andy Cochrane, however, was contacted (Cochrane, email, December 2015). Results were yet to be published but he contended that there was still uncertainty as to the effectiveness of reablement. The main issue at that time was the lack of robust studies, in particular those that employed quantitative methods (comparative), with only two meeting the eligibility criteria: one in Australia and the other in Norway. Essentially both Regan, Wells and Foreman (2009) and Cochrane and colleagues (2013) describe reablement as a programme of multifaceted approaches; this may include exercises, behavioural changes, education, environmental adjustments/adaptations, provision of equipment by way of compensation for illness or disability, and use of local/community-based resources.

Since its introduction in 2006, the Department of Health's Care Services Efficiency Delivery (CSED) Programme has evaluated the progress in developing home care reablement services in England. The setup of the CSED resulted from the Gershon Review in 2004 which was conducted, in brief, to 'release resources to the front line'. The analysis phase was between September 2004 and February 2005 (DH 2007a) and its purpose was to maximise available resources and ultimately benefit people through better delivery of services. This was a collaborative venture by the CSED alongside councils with social service responsibility (CSSRs).

Leading definitions for reablement in the UK can be found in reports by the Care Services Efficiency Delivery (CSED 2010a) programme. The earliest however was coined by Kent and colleagues (2000) who name reablement by type as:

> Services for people with poor physical or mental health

> To help them accommodate their illness (or condition) by learning or relearning the skills necessary for daily living

Arguably, this definition is somewhat limited. It fails to take into account the philosophical stance of reablement which suggests that a somewhat radical change in the provision of paid care needs to take place. Wood and Salter (2012) also contend that other definitions offer broader considerations such as social abilities as well as making more explicit what they and others (CSED 2009; COT 2013; Skelton 2013) refer to, as the 'enablement ethos' (philosophy). A range of innovative practice alternatives are possible when these are considered, as well as a move away from a reductionist approach ('pragmatist versus structuralist'; see Chapter 2). This is, however, fraught with contention due to the very different structure of main stream services, and the need for more contact time for support workers, to facilitate people's reablement effectively (Miller 2014). Another definition of reablement by the CSED in 2009, and the result of a longitudinal study, makes further reference to the desired philosophy:

> Reablement can be described as an 'approach' or a 'philosophy' within home care services – one which aims to help people 'do things for themselves', rather than 'having things done for them'.
>
> (NEIEP 2010, p. 5)

Returning to the structure of mainstream services there is evidence across the literature on reablement that there is a blurring of models. These include intermediate care, rehabilitation and reablement and to some extent, preventative services. Essentially, people often find themselves somewhat confused as to what service they are receiving and this aspect was discussed in more depth in Chapter 2. The move away from traditional, often in-house, home care services has been widespread. Essentially this may help in reducing a culture of dependency with a focus towards more autonomous and community living. Just as significantly, it is also one route to reducing the long-term cost of social care. To this extent, it is important to understand that reablement, as discussed here, is considered a philosophy for some or just a process for others.

Following the release of the *Putting people first* white paper (DH 2007), many councils began to introduce reablement services with the aim of reducing and/or delaying the cost of long-term home care to councils. In addition, by working with older people in this manner, there is a positive impact on the delay for, or need for, people to leave their home and go into a care home setting. Glendinning and Newbronner (2008) suggest that adopting a reablement approach to service provision can delay the need for ongoing home care by as much as 12 months. The subsequent evidence, however, five years later, of improved quality of life is seen as having far greater value (Glendinning 2013). Service provision formats are varied in terms of who provides it. This might be in the context of the make-up/skill mix of the teams, or whether it is social care with links to NHS partners, or indeed, terms of reablement location. It should be community-based with services provided in the person's own home, but can also be provided in extra care housing type settings as a 'step-up' approach before returning to independent living. Extra care settings include sheltered housing or assisted living apartments.

Sanderson and Lewis (2012), much like NEIEP (2010), allude to a reablement ethos, describing it as a journey rather than a service and one that is applicable to all users – not just older people. With this said there is a danger that local authority reablement interventions are leading to the service being viewed as just for older people – rather than for all. This may be due to the volume of older people who were once assessed on their critical and substantial needs under Fair Access to Care Services (FACS) (see the section 'Model two: Intake and assessment reablement service') and the consequence of an ageing population with chronic long-term needs.

From a delivery perspective, it is argued that occupational therapists' (OT) unique skills and training in rehabilitation, recovery and enabling, makes their involvement essential to the success of reablement services (Skelton 2013). While the idea of a reablement approach is relatively new to home care services, it is one that has always been core to OT practice and in particular its overarching ethos. These practitioners are ideally suited to provide expertise not only in the development of reablement services but also in its delivery:

> A strong priority should be placed on the involvement of occupational therapy particularly in the planning of the service and supervision of reablement support staff.
>
> (SCIE 2011a; Skelton 2013; Health and Social Care Board 2015)

While their assessment skills also make them best placed to identify potential reablement goals with people, OTs' input in reablement services varies across the country, in both the level and the timeliness of their interventions. OTs have long since recognised the health benefits of staying engaged in daily living tasks. With this in mind, it can be argued that they are also key in the establishment of reablement services but also in terms of best trainers for support worker development.

Reablement is a successful service when the goals are set by the individual. Traditionally, home care has often revolved around meal times, linking personal care and toileting to these call times (morning, midday, evenings and during the night). Reablement is at its best when it is not only flexible in the time of the visits but also the nature of the tasks being done – not solely revolving around personal care tasks or meal preparation – but the wider gambit of activities of daily living (ADL) that are important to an individual. Evidence shows that by ensuring goals are individualised, and that a person-centred approach is adopted, motivation can increase and reablement thus has a higher success rate (Newton 2012; Wilde and Glendinning 2012).

No discussion of reablement services can take place without recognition of the **social model of disability** (Rabiee and Glendinning 2011) in which the individual's needs are looked at holistically (see Chapter 4). A social work/social care perspective acknowledges the importance of empowering individuals to regain control and autonomy and so the reablement model sits very well within this framework. Limitations to reablement, however, and which are discussed in more depth later on, include:

> Challenges in transforming social care and developing a nationwide approach

> Start-up costs and issues with retraining the whole home care workforce

> Problems when care is transferred back to 'conventional' home care services

Interlinks is a Europe-wide resource that aims to improve long-term person-centred care for older people. The limitations above are very much reflected in a summary on the website with a message asking for more research and monitoring to: '... gain further insight into how best to deliver re-ablement services and how services impact on different user groups' (Interlinks, n.d.).

We now consider four models of reablement that have been developed in health and social care services: model one looks at a social care model of reablement following hospital discharge; model two is an intake and assessment approach based on a local authority in the north-west of England; model three has an integrated focus; while model four considers future models of reablement.

Models of reablement service provision

Model one: Hospital discharge service

The focus of any reablement service is to help the individual to regain skills (Sanderson and Lewis 2012), and in particular the social care model is an ideal framework, as it draws on empowerment and enablement principles. A hospital discharge service includes, as one of its aims, a drive to reduce risk of readmission to hospital. Consequently, care planning will include health-related needs, but despite the rhetoric, it is not so much concerned with social care issues. Following the introduction of Clinical Commissioning Groups (CCGs) in 2013 in the UK, reablement services may become pivotal in providing a seamless system of integration between **secondary health** and social care. Furthermore, this care planning must include a determined approach towards prevention, anticipation and supported self-reliance. When hospital treatment is no longer required and the patient's discharge is pending, the aim should be to return him or her home as soon as possible, while forward planning to minimise risk of readmission.

With the hospital discharge model, it is likely that two of the criteria for referral to a reablement service (aside from being medically stable) is a health need (often multiple and complex), **capacity to consent** and rehabilitation potential. Once the person is discharged into the community the aim of the reablement service is to promote and encourage autonomy in everyday living. The referral criteria for this kind of service therefore includes a condition or conditions that no longer require hospital intervention; understanding of the concept of reablement; and motivation to accept and work with the reablement team towards autonomy. Some services will not take on those with mental health issues and others have a sole focus on, for example, dementia or Alzheimer's disease. Reablement is available in most instances for adults from the age of 18 years, but is primarily used by people aged 60 years and over. It is offered to those who would otherwise:

➤ Remain in hospital when there is no longer a health need

➤ Be discharged home with either full state-funded or private (formal) care

The outcome of both scenarios above would result in loss of autonomy, increased dependence and quality of life could be compromised. At yet another level it incurs greater costs to social care services.

Reablement services in general are finite in nature, usually short-term for up to six weeks, and people are generally not charged within this timescale. Offering reablement services to people at a time when they are keen to return home from hospital may be mistimed. This is because once they are at home their original commitment to the goals agreed might change, or they might not be well enough to work on them and require a period of resettlement at home first. A better use of limited resources might be for a supported discharge scheme for a short period after leaving hospital, followed by a community-based assessment for reablement services. This would be to regain previous levels of function in the home or alternatively identify if a maintenance scheme may be more appropriate.

A person-centred approach

Reablement requires a person-centred focus. Needs are assessed but in consultation with the person, much the same as in Scenario 3.1 (see p. 83) describing Alice's experience. This then results in an individually tailored scheme of care. The social model of disability emphasises the importance of empowerment and capacity building and this notion should underpin all approaches to care (SCIE 2012a). Even in instances where capacity to consent may be limited (such as for those with dementia), it is still possible to empower people – regardless of their disability, impairment or cognitive difficulties – and by standing back and encouraging and promoting autonomy this facilitates 'taking control'. The person's motivation alongside realistic expectation are essential. They therefore need to be able to understand the difference between traditional home care and reablement. There is little benefit to providing a reablement service if the person does not understand or is not motivated to do things for themselves. With appropriate staff training and an understanding of how to 'motivate to participate', it is possible to engage people so they can see the health benefits and positive impact of increased autonomy in daily living tasks.

The following is a response by an interviewee on her uncertainty about reablement prior to discharge:

> I didn't understand all of it … I was just told I'd get a carer coming in, in the morning, to come and help me get washed and dressed.
> (Quoted in Wilde and Glendinning 2012, p. 586)

Interestingly, the metaphorical term 'standing back' is quite literally a balance between allowing someone to fail and taking over completely. It is an integral skill of all OTs who have a specialist understanding of ADL. This is their distinction from all other professions allied to medicine. Core academic and practice training involves, among other subjects, kinesiology and ergonomics relevant to occupation or, as discussed in Chapter 1, ADL. This is why OT assessment is so important in the context of reablement, and why intervention needs to be intelligently considered, allowing the person sufficient time before a decision on capability or competence is made. It is also another factor as to why OTs are key in the training of support workers.

Scenario 3.1 The impact of hospital discharge with and without a reablement package

Alice had been in hospital for five weeks, with a planned discharge for reablement services once she was determined medically stable. Unfortunately, before the reablement support could take place Alice had a setback and returned to hospital the same day. She then spent another three weeks in hospital and during this time it was decided that she had no rehabilitation potential. Alice was subsequently discharged with a high level of maintenance care because she was reliant on support, for almost all personal activities of daily living (PADL) and all domestic activities of daily living (DADL).

Three weeks after discharge Alice was assessed by an OT in her home environment. The outcome of this assessment was that she had improved to such an extent that she was now an excellent candidate for reablement. A common and frequent scenario is missing the potential for rehabilitation or a lack of signposting while the person is in the hospital setting. At times and because of limited and stretched resources, including staff, it is sometimes more pragmatic and considered safer to reinstate prior provision or a new scheme. This is the consequence also of discharges which have occurred as a result of bed shortages.

At home Alice was keen to be able to walk safely but had to use a standing aid. She wanted to regain her previous level of independence with this prior to her hospital admission. Reablement goals were agreed with the OT, and support staff started working in partnership with her on a regular daily basis. Alice responded positively and quite soon she was able to walk with supervision in her home environment. She also reported feeling a sense of achievement and well-being as she was being encouraged to take care of her personal care needs. During the reablement period, with comprehensive feedback from staff as well as input from a physiotherapist, it was agreed that Alice might be presenting with symptoms similar to those of Parkinson's disease. Her GP was contacted and intervention/treatment ensued. The situation was then jointly managed by community health services and the local authority reablement service. Consequently, Alice's mobility improved, the result of which negated the need for supervision and there were no further hospital admissions for another three years.

Model two: Intake and assessment reablement service

Some local authorities began to use reablement services as an intake and assessment service for ongoing social care needs (Wood and Salter 2012).

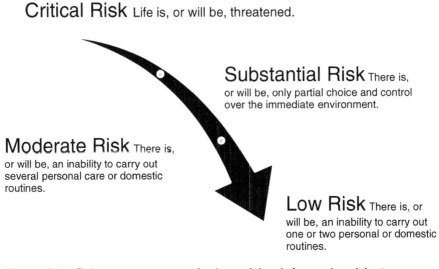

Critical Risk Life is, or will be, threatened.

Substantial Risk There is, or will be, only partial choice and control over the immediate environment.

Moderate Risk There is, or will be, an inability to carry out several personal care or domestic routines.

Low Risk There is, or will be, an inability to carry out one or two personal or domestic routines.

Figure 3.1   Fair access to care criteria explained: Assessing risks to independence
Adapted from SCIE (2013)

These services applied the national FACs criteria to establish an individual's eligibility for services. FACs was introduced in 2003 (and updated seven years later) as a process or framework to assess levels of need or risk to independence over time. It was devised as a fairer system for providing support with the aim of providing transparency from one borough to the next (DH 2010). Only those individuals with needs above a certain level would have been able to access a reablement service under FACs criteria. In order to meet this criterion, an individual generally would have had critical or substantial risks to their independence (see Figure 3.1).

The implementation of the Care Act (DH 2014a, b), together with a more preventative agenda adopted by local authorities, aims to defer the point at which people reach crisis point, and introduce a wider approach to assessment. It is meant to be preventative and integrative in nature including both carer and person cared for. In addition, it requires local authorities to collaborate, co-operate and integrate more with health and housing services. The criteria in FACs did not offer equity because many individuals struggled greatly even if they only had moderate or low-risk needs. The assessment and eligibility process map by SCIE (2015) illustrates the Care Act 2014 (DH 2014a). See https://www.scie.org.uk/care-act-2014/assessment-and-eligibility/process-map/. It also demonstrates how a wider and more integrative approach to assessment can be preventative and more equitable.

Referrals to an intake and assessment service are mainly from the community such as via a GP, social worker (SW), neighbour or family member. Community nurses involved in health assessment and interventions can also identify if a person is medically stable and whether they might benefit from reablement. This would lead to an initial assessment of the person's suitability for reablement, and to determine whether the person understands reablement, and that they are motivated to try a new approach. They will have goals that they wish to achieve through reablement support. People who are unlikely to benefit from this service are screened out (Glendinning 2013) and redirected to other services. These instances were discussed earlier.

This model may be seen as having replaced traditional social services home care provision, involving to a greater extent 'hands-on' assistance with PADL and DADL. In some instances, reablement, which is offered in a local authority, may have been developed alongside its existing home care services. The result of this type of 'bolt-on' service results, more often than not, in a lack of adequate training for support staff who are used to 'doing for' people rather than standing back. A traditional home care service that offers reablement might then be considered as one that pays lip service to a new approach and has a name change but little else. The result is that less time is spent on promoting and encouraging people to return to, or maintain their autonomy in, ADL. So arguably, transferring a traditional home care service to a reablement service is not as effective in the long term, unless support staff receive adequate training. Potentially the risk is there for inadequately trained staff to undo the reablement progress made (Pilkington 2008). This is not exclusively about how to approach facilitation of ADL with people, but also about developing their understanding that reablement has an entirely different ethos to traditional home care. Some organisations, with this add-on to existing provision, find that staff have difficulties in understanding their role to encourage and promote confidence while supporting an individual to regain his or her lost skills.

Social care organisations must, out of necessity, review the way they provide services in the long term to people who are living at home autonomously. More importantly, reablement services work to maximum efficiency and avoid at all costs becoming a temporary 'patch-up' solution. Many local authorities have taken the view that the statutory responsibility for providing long-term home care does not have to be provided by an 'in-house' care staff, but rather can be met by existing private care agencies. This can be a positive move but is dependent on effective forethought, planning and preparation. Local authority adult services are usually responsible for providing or commissioning this type of service. It is likely that the previous home care service provided by the local authority will have transferred to a reablement-only service or been tendered out to a third-sector provider. There are positives and negatives to this approach that affect both the person and the worker.

When using existing home care workers, local authorities will need to retrain workers to undertake reablement tasks – an area that was explored in Chapter 2. Reablement requires the home care support worker to do more than stand by and watch the person, as they need to offer support, guidance and encouragement as well as an awareness of when it is appropriate to step in and assist the individual. The ability to stand back was discussed earlier in this chapter entitled 'A person Centred Approach' p. 83. Staff in general and anecdotally home care support workers can find it difficult to switch between a traditional care role and a reablement role (Crank, conference 2013). Without appropriate training, however, staff can feel ill-equipped and lack confidence to use the same enabling approach with all people, not just those receiving a 'reablement package of care' (Newton 2012; SCIE 2011b). Therefore, there is a need for workers to adapt to a new way of working. This brings us back to the enablement ethos or philosophy of reablement which was discussed earlier (see p. 78, NEIEP 2010).

Added to this, work patterns and employer expectations about time and cost are rooted in traditional daily interactions and behaviours. This means that workers are used to doing things 'for' people and often feel they 'don't have time' to stand back and enable them. Clearly job satisfaction creates a good working environment and motivation plays a big part. One service in the north-west of England is testament to this after a dramatic change in mind-set towards reablement and in the approach of service providers. They were greatly encouraged when they witnessed the positive outcomes. Staff members and service users reap the rewards of a reablement approach (Mickel 2010). It works at different levels. Support staff, however, benefit from having at least NVQ level 2 or 3 as a starting point. This may allow for better comprehension of different ways of working (tasks) and it may also help to a certain extent in understanding the emphasis on a 'hands-off' approach. This is supported by SCIE (2012b) and the United Kingdom Homecare Association who acknowledge:

> There needs to be a significant shift in the culture of working – which some care workers will adapt to more easily than others – for reablement to happen.

The York study (Glendinning 2013) found that staff with less experience in traditional home care were able to adapt more easily to this type of work. There is a view that new staff who have not previously undertaken traditional home care tasks are better suited to the role (SCIE 2011a, 2012c).

Example 1: An intake and assessment service

An example of this model includes a local authority in the north-west of England. This authority established a reablement service in 2009, tailored for people who met FACS criteria and were deemed to have substantial or critical needs, requiring carer support at home. The service was to be one of an all-inclusive nature. Those who were on an end-of-life pathway or care plan (terminal illness) and people who had significant cognitive impairment – meaning that learning/relearning would not be possible – would not benefit. As mentioned earlier, some reablement services are specifically tailored for people with dementia (see p. 81).

Service provision and appropriateness of referral is also determined through selection criteria being met by the person, and only those judged to benefit from the process are selected (DH 2007a). The nature of selection into reablement services – significantly – determines the volume of the people that use them, and the outcome of the service provision is reliant on staffing numbers, expertise (or understanding) and level of interdisciplinary professional support. It is argued here that success is also dependent on how well staff work interprofessionally and from a partnership working perspective – to the inclusion of the person and family. The term interprofessional is used here and given to mean that the people from different professions not only work and communicate with each other, but also learn from and about each other. Other aspects relevant to interprofessional working are discussed in Chapter 5.

Alongside this particular reablement service, the local authority continued to operate a 'traditional style' of domiciliary home care. This is useful because once the reablement period concludes a financial assessment should take place. If required, long-term formal care can be set up (if necessary), which then remains with the 'in-house' service or alternatively with an external provider (agency). This is critical as sometimes a person may develop autonomy in a number of activities but still require formal care as discussed in Chapters 1 and 2. The co-existence of the two services using the same workforce became a factor in how successful the reablement service was at this time. It became evident that there was a conflict for staff between 'reablement' and 'maintenance' (or long-term care) service users. Support staff found it difficult to switch between the two, and did not feel they had the skills to be able to use the reablement approach with all service users regardless of their named support package.

The service developed over time to include more mandatory training specifically in reablement alongside one-to-one OT support for home care support workers. The ethos of reablement became more and more embedded in the way the staff worked. In addition, there was a division at a later date of the two work streams. Traditional home care was transferred to the private sector, leaving only the 'in-house' reablement service. There was also staff redeployment; those wishing to continue with traditional home care were no longer employed by the council. This change of both staffing and services meant that a complete focus could be given to reablement alongside appropriate training for the much smaller dedicated workforce.

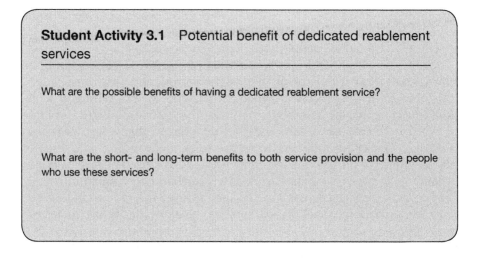

Student Activity 3.1   Potential benefit of dedicated reablement services

What are the possible benefits of having a dedicated reablement service?

What are the short- and long-term benefits to both service provision and the people who use these services?

Model three: An integrated model

The social care policy driver for subsequent reablement services came from the National Service Framework for Older People (NSFOP) (DH 2001). Standard 3 of the NSFOP introduced the concept of intermediate care in which the focus was on providing care either in the home environment which would be hospital at home (acute care) or through supported discharge with a need for medical management from nurses and therapeutic input. Locations for intermediate care also include community hospitals or contracts to nursing homes where often one floor is dedicated to the service. Intermediate care helps prevent admission to hospital and promotes autonomy though effective rehabilitation, but it also facilitates early discharge from hospital at a time when the person is considered medically stable. A key driver of these services was for them to operate between health and social care services (DH 2002) and to focus on active rehabilitation.

Intermediate care is defined as 'a range of integrated services to promote faster recovery from illness, prevent unnecessary acute hospital admission and premature admission to long-term residential care, support timely discharge from hospital and maximise independent living' (CSED 2010b, p. 1). The CSED goes on to define further criteria for intermediate care as:

> Targeted at people who would otherwise have an unnecessary prolonged hospital stay

> Based on comprehensive assessment, usually in hospital, resulting in a structured care plan that usually involves active therapy, treatment or opportunity for recovery

> Planned outcome for maximising independence and typically enabling people to return to living at home

> Usually time-limited, not normally more than six weeks, but frequently as little as one to two weeks

> Involves cross-professional working with a single assessment, single professional record and shared protocols

(CSED 2010b, p. 2)

In summary, the best way to describe intermediate care is as a 'half-way home' service and this is the term CSED used in 2010 to denote this difference from reablement (CSED 2010b). Increasingly, with the push for integrated health and social care services over the past ten years, councils have sought effective routes and services to help to avoid costly hospital admissions. Reablement services fall nicely into this framework, combining with discharge teams, hospital at home services, OT and physiotherapy (PT) interventions with a multidisciplinary (MDT) approach to keeping people at home. With the focus of reablement being restorative in nature, it makes sense that a reablement home support package could be commissioned to aid someone back to health, for example following a fall. Falls are a frequent cause of hospital admission for older people (NICE 2013). Once in hospital their discharge can often be delayed, more often due to cancellation of current care and sourcing new care schemes. To some extent the inevitable deterioration in physical ability, stamina and overall well-being is also attributed to lethargy brought on by hospital stays. It is better for the person to be supported in their own home if there is no medical need preventing them to do so. In this, their familiar environment, the person can work on regaining not only their confidence but their strength in daily living tasks. It is thus critical that the hospital team work together closely so that all eventualities are addressed. More often than not an environmental home visit, including at least two of the hospital-based MDT (OT, PT, SW and if necessary nurse) assists greatly with discharge planning. This is particularly the case for reablement.

From a policy perspective, local joint health and well-being strategies (DH 2012) continue to be integrated within services across health and social care. This has been supported with considerable financial backing to develop reablement services. Effective reablement, intermediate care and post-discharge support mean that people returning home after a stay in hospital should have a temporary support plan that helps them to regain their autonomy. This ensures they are not pressured into decisions about long-term support at a time when they are not well enough or in the right place to make those decisions. There is clearly a need for joined-up communication between reablement and intermediate care services. This is in order to avoid the current duplication of services and to ensure a seamless support system for people to achieve their full potential after a period of illness or injury (DH 2012).

At this point it is important to reiterate and make clear the distinctions between intermediate care and reablement. The main function of intermediate care is to prevent hospital admissions, speed up hospital discharges and prevent or delay admission to long-term residential/nursing care. Reablement on the other hand is sought at a point where previously a 'care package' would have been considered necessary, or is already in place. While reablement services often have quick links to therapists, particularly OTs, intermediate care services are often led by clinicians: nurses, OTs, physiotherapists. A number of services across the UK are linking these two service approaches in a more integrated way.

Step-up/step-down service provision relates in general to intermediate care services that can be provided either in a person's own home or in a 24-hour supported environment that is outside of acute hospital settings. The idea behind this is that people are provided with a higher level of support than they currently receive to prevent them being admitted to hospital, or to speed up discharge from hospital. This form of intermediate care is delivered in a variety of ways and is associated with many different terms – hospital at home services, early supported discharge services, rapid response services, interdisciplinary rehabilitation teams; even reablement teams have been described in terms of 'post-discharge support' to name but a few. Often these intermediate care services are based around quick access to OT and/or PT interventions. One council in the north-west of England has taken this a step further and has adopted a pilot service that enables rapid access to domiciliary care, the aim being to avoid hospital admission by providing timely care in the home environment. This may then be followed by a period of reablement, when the person's health is more stable, to enable them to work towards their previous level of autonomy. Alternatively, it enables prompt discharge from hospital prior to setting up a reablement service or indeed formal care support.

Model four: Reablement in the future

Outsourcing reablement home care

With ever increasing pressure on councils to find efficiencies and manage demand, outsourcing reablement services may become a more frequent consideration in the future. At present a fairly small number of councils (20 out of 149) have taken this approach to reablement provision (Gerald Pilkington Associates 2011). Most reablement services originally developed from in-house home care services and many councils have opted to keep reablement as an in-house service. This is in part because reablement interventions require close management and supervision, and staff training, resulting in high hourly costs which are not often viable for independent providers.

Councils have also maintained reablement as an in-house service due to concerns that outsourcing creates perverse incentives. The theory is that a private provider has no business incentive to improve someone's independence and reduce their care package because it would reduce their own core business. Councils and private providers have adopted different approaches to overcoming this problem. Some care agencies have used an alternative business model, only accepting referrals for reablement clients – as opposed to basing their business on providing 'maintenance care'. Councils who have outsourced reablement have dealt with potential problems through outcomes-based commissioning. Traditionally councils have invested in training of staff to reasonably high levels (although in some instances quality could be better), thereby creating a valuable resource, not necessarily mirrored in private care agencies where there has been little or no training on reablement approaches to care. An integral part of successful outsourced reablement provision is training of staff – councils are then faced with a decision as to their involvement in this and the cost element associated with ongoing training. If adequate training however is not provided the result may be poorer outcomes for individuals and higher costs to social care. Three main models for outsourcing reablement have emerged:

1. *Creating a local authority trading company and transferring the reablement service*. This allows a level of strategic control, while retaining the knowledge and skill base of the service, but at the same time retaining some of the risks and costs associated with reablement services.

2. *Transferring the service to a social enterprise company*. As in point 1, the skills and knowledge will be retained but the council would have a reduced level of control of the service to the same level as any other contracted care provider.

3. *Outsourcing to the independent sector.* Transferring all the risk and associated costs to the external agency. The knowledge and skill base will be there initially but there is no guarantee that this will continue at the same level. Councils would lose control and influence over the service as with any contracted care provider and would have to have strict commissioning contracts in place that are outcome-focused.

As with all outsourced services, councils need to ensure contractual arrangements are thorough and have some way of monitoring the service they are providing. This can be complicated with a fully outsourced arrangement unless there are proper reporting mechanisms in place.

Service provision in adult social care has altered greatly in recent years. From a once cohesive 'in-house' home care service, where the relationship between the person and the social worker (SW) and frontline carer was a long-standing and effective one, to a seemingly much more fragmented service with outsourced care agencies (Robb 2013).

Accessing services

In the same council in the north-west of England, access to service provision has developed to provide a more preventative assessment approach. Fox and colleagues (2012) described the need for an altered community care process that triggers early assessment which enables risk and planning to be carried out at a more timely stage, that is, before the person has reached crisis point. This has been incorporated into an initial assessment being carried out by OTs prior to any social care services being allocated. It is widely recognised that activity analysis and assessment of functional ability is at the core of OT thus making these practitioners ideally placed to become involved at this early stage. Not only is this advantageous to the client who is seen more quickly, but they are then assessed and directed to the most appropriate service without delay. This approach has meant that if reablement is seen as suitable for the person, the OT is able to immediately start the service, setting appropriate goals with the person for the reablement staff to follow. This targeted approach means a higher success rate for clients who are appropriately placed with reablement, it also enables the avoidance and/or delay of long-term social care by compensating for any difficulties with equipment, technique or approach to ADL tasks (see Chapter 1). In addition, this approach frees up social workers to engage in the more complex social care case management.

Student Activity 3.2 Long-term conditions and/or learning disabilities

Discuss how service provision could be improved for people with long-term conditions such as clinical depression. Think through how a short-term reablement service might work for these people.

Consider reablement interventions for older people with learning disabilities. What might be the approach here and is there anyone in particular you would want to have on your team?

Not only are councils changing the way they deliver home care, some are also changing the way they deliver reablement. Outsourcing to private companies is becoming more and more common. In addition, reducing the number of social workers by improving access to services and delaying and/ or preventing individuals reaching crisis point alters the type of service provided. Traditionally social workers were involved with families and people in general when they had reached crisis point. With the advent of personalisation, stronger community support, third-sector support and reablement services, people and their families are supported to prevent reaching crisis point.

On the other hand, one could argue that councils are being short-sighted. The question arises whether reducing the numbers of qualified social workers, bearing in mind the increasing numbers of older people in the coming years, is an effective long-term strategy. There is an assumption that the social worker's remit is only assessment of need and support for people to access services – rather than a much broader role in adult social care (Samuel 2012).

Social reablement

One major issue, which is identified at several points throughout this book, is the issue of isolation and/or loneliness. In the context of reablement this is parallel to abandonment for some individuals when a six-week reablement service withdraws. The focus on what seems to be essentially daily living tasks, such as personal and domestic care, fails to address 'being' and 'belonging' in the community. There is a tendency to return to the didactic focus on personalisation and person-centred care whenever calls for change are made in health and social care (personalisation and person-centred care addressed in greater depth; chapters 2 and 4). Didactic from this perspective refers to the idea that reablement team members consider that they already practise in this person-centred way and that they are holistic – taking all factors into account. A vital and reasonable argument, however, is that reablement has the potential to address far more pressing needs than PADL and DADL. A lack of contact with family, friends or the community oftentimes equates to social isolation and this is known as a risk factor for loneliness. In a situation of isolation, you could have several visits from family members or indeed formal carers but still be lonely. Here it is more about the quality of the relationship that is the defining point. Age UK identify in a major review of the literature on loneliness and social isolation (Davidson 2014) that a sense of disconnection with others can lead to: '[a] profound impact on physical and mental health, and quality of life' (p. 3).

> *Like geese whose V formation goes unnoticed; we sometimes ignore the value of relationships, forgetting that meaningful daily interaction brings health to body and mind.*

The social model of disability, despite recent criticisms, does help in identifying barriers in society that potentially exclude the individual, or make it difficult for them to fully participate in local communities. By identifying barriers, it is then possible to support the individual to be able to participate. The reablement models discussed in this chapter can address such barriers or functional difficulties, but the primary aim is to do this by reducing the need for formal or informal care support. By enabling the person to participate autonomously in society and daily living, care is reduced or at best withdrawn. The by-product of this of course is that social independence for many older adults is transient; there comes a time when these activities become more difficult. At that point the risk is that social needs become neglected if the leisure activities chosen to address, this need are not based in day centres or other group settings. For most, if there is little or limited contact with the 'outside world', the risk of falling, increasing ill health or hospital admission, is far greater. So therefore, social reablement needs to take a prospective approach, so that on withdrawing a service, a fixed point in time is agreed in order to do a review. The question arises here as to how many of the reablement services across the country are able to do this, given finite resources. It is also difficult to assess how well other services link into reablement: whether there is shared electronic records, for example, or sound knowledge of referral criteria and what reablement can realistically achieve within locality budgets.

Reablement like any other service is result-focused which is important in the justification of interventions and economy of scale. If we are outcomes-driven, which is the case in most health and social care services, perhaps we should be paying more attention to social needs – but not in a 'catch-all' scenario such as day care or centres. If we truly adopt the ideas of personalisation and of goal planning in co-participation with people, it makes sense to place additional emphasis on increasing well-being through 'meaningful' social activities. Activities such as going to a local luncheon club, going out to the pub on occasion or attending a film appreciation group through, for example, the Third Age University:

> The U3A taught me things I have missed along life's way.
>
> (Quoted in U3A 2014, p. 3)

Another aspect that is gaining momentum is the ideas taken from the discipline of positive psychology. This discipline considers that all individuals want to engage in meaningful lives and occupations in the pursuit of happiness. So instead of focusing on what is wrong, as traditional psychology does, positive psychology considers what makes life worth living – in other words, our well-being. Inspired by several initiatives and think tanks such as the New Economics Foundation, there is now a greater emphasis on well-being – which is not related to wealth or 'gross domestic product'. One such initiative, held in a town in the north-west of England and aptly named the 'Festival of Wellbeing' (The Atkinson 2014), included in its list of activities and lectures:

➤ Principles and technique of mindfulness (see Chapter 2)

➤ Zumba, Tai Chi as well as chair-based exercise, cycling and walking

➤ Impact of creativity on health – Merseycare's Recovery College, 'Creative Alternatives'

➤ 'Good Food, Good Mood' – healthy eating promotions

➤ Befriending 'Speed chats'

➤ Sea Change Tour – the changing face of the north-west's coast

➤ A pop-up of a 1950s living room designed to encourage positive reminiscence

The activities were for all ages but many of the events were clearly aimed at older people. A local line dancing group, The Oakland Mavericks, are based in a small community in Thingwall, and also at two other sites on the Wirral. The sessions are led by a retired couple, Nick and Alison. Member ages range from the youngest at fifty, to the oldest at eighty-seven. The majority who attend are over seventy-five and at last count there were approximately eighty members. Many have long term conditions, some quite limiting, yet... they come every week or even twice-weekly. When watching the group dance, it seems as if they are 'lost in the moment'; an aspect that Csikszentmihalyi (1990) coined as 'flow'. There is a sense of real belonging and community that transcends just dancing. Mistaken moves and steps turn into laughter and there is an air of joviality at each gathering. Individuals offer support to each other when one person becomes unwell or is in crisis caring for a partner. Nick and Alison raise money most weeks for a range of charities. This gives the attendees a sense of 'giving back' to others, a unity in spirit and importantly - purpose. Some drive but also fetch members who struggle with local transport due to balance or difficulties walking distances. No one in the group needs to feel lonely or isolated and when dancing they are moving, increasing their dexterity, but most importantly laughing.

Naturally, not everyone would find these activities pleasurable or, if they did, be able to get to them. It would be simplistic therefore to also assume that every older adult would want to participate. Some of the issues that may hinder this, however, are fairly easy to pinpoint:

> Money for transport (why not pool resources or a fund within a locality?)

> Type of transport (buses with assistive technology for people with balance/walking difficulties?)

> Location distance (why not organise according to locality – SMART technology?)

> Reduced stamina and mobility (why not invite less able people to each other's homes?)

> Fluctuating and unpredictable health (why not keep in touch – SMART technology?)

> Access to a telephone or indeed the outside world

If we consider that, at this time, the emphasis for the better part in intermediate and rehabilitative services is more often centred on primary needs – such as personal care and management of domestic ADL – it is clear that social needs are a widely neglected and under-represented area.

FACT 3.1

> 17% of older people are in contact with family, friends and neighbours less than once a week and 11% are in contact less than once a month

> Over half (51%) of all people aged 75 and over live alone

> Two-fifths of all older people (about 3.9 million) say the television is their main company

▶

◀

➣ 63% of adults aged 52 or over who have been widowed, and 51% of the same group who are separated or divorced, report feeling lonely some of the time or often

➣ 59% of adults aged over 52 who report poor health say they feel lonely some of the time or often, compared to 21% who say they are in excellent health

➣ A higher percentage of women than men report feeling lonely some of the time or often.

Sources: **Data taken from several sources, including Age UK (2014); Campaign to End Loneliness (2015); Beaumont (2013); Victor et al. (2003)**

Six reviews of qualitative studies since 1984 identified the main strategies for reducing loneliness. These were (1) improving social skills, (2) enhancing social support, (3) increasing opportunities for social interaction, and (4) addressing maladaptive social cognition. The efficacy, however, of these interventions was questioned. Better, more rigorous research was needed. To that extent Masi and colleagues (2011) carried out a quantitative meta-analysis. Out of the 928 articles only 50 were considered, as the others failed to meet all the inclusion criteria. They concluded that all the interventions listed above were successful (in varying degrees) in reducing loneliness, but that interventions attempting to alter maladaptive social cognition were most effective. Arguably, the environment should be taken into consideration alongside support to find out what is available locally and of interest to a person. It is also argued here that a person who has lived into older adulthood does not require assistance in 'improving social skills' as identified by Masi and colleagues (2011) in their strategy review. The idea of maladaptive social cognition is also questionable unless of course the individual has a mental health difficulty.

Student Activity 3.3   Improving connections and social lives

Aside from the activities from the Festival of Wellbeing, what others might an older individual want to engage in?

Think about what you might like to do in your later years if you were living alone.

➣ Enjoy a meal prepared, cooked and eaten with others?

➣ Going to the theatre with people the same age as you (or not) who share a similar interest?

Importantly, all those involved in either developing or improving existing reablement services must think with foresight – with co-production in mind. This was discussed in Chapter 2. Beresford (2015) warns, however, that the '[m]ore confident and assertive service users are often unpopular among those organising involvement activities and dismissed as "the usual suspects"'. Wilde and Glendinning (2012, p. 583) conclude in their study that if we can gain a better understanding of service user perspectives, reablement services should be more effective. This comes nonetheless with the proviso that this must be in terms of service users' own priorities and definitions of autonomy. If our aim is to be truly person-centred, and we want to demonstrate a concerted move towards genuine personalisation, our first aim should be to overcome these tensions.

Conclusion

The aim of this chapter has been to give the reader an insight into models of reablement service provision, starting with the hospital discharge model, moving on to a more community-based intake and assessment model, followed by a more integrated approach to reablement and concluding with some examples and discussion points for the future of reablement service provision. For the purposes of clarity these models have been outlined separately but in reality there is often a blurring of models dependent upon the person's journey through the health and social care system and how the organisations are set up around them. A person's journey in health and social care is never linear but is dynamic, changing and adapting according to their needs.

Although this chapter has intended to give the reader an outline of models of reablement service provision, it is by no means exhaustive. Reablement service provision is variable across the country depending on a multitude of factors: geography, rural versus urban areas, population numbers, services already in place, budgetary factors, and development of integration plans across health and social care. There are also significant differences internationally.

Wilde and Glendinning (2012) argue that while reablement works well for those with conditions that lend well to the preventative nature of step-up/step-down health services and possible avoidance of hospital admissions, there is a further sector of the population where long-term, progressive conditions would not benefit from the same 'preventative' services, when there is a deterioration in health – whether temporarily or long term. Every individual has their own unique set of circumstances, coping mechanisms and motivation. A reablement scheme is an option even if short-term illness develops alongside long-term conditions, but sometimes a person simply needs some 'hands-on' support. The benefits of being flexible in these situations are important but an adequate review a few weeks or months after formal care is in place will always be useful. Pitts and colleagues (2011) suggest that reablement requires a different approach and one that assimilates person-centred practice so that it is more holistic and not narrow. We need to be aware of individuals' inter-dependence with services but also acknowledge when they can return to playing an autonomous role again when the time is right. Not every-one will benefit from reablement services, as Manthorpe (2011) notes in a discussion about a study conducted in 2010 by the University of York (Glendinning 2013). This research looked at the long-term impact of reablement, concluding that targeted services may be more successful in meeting long-term need as not everyone will benefit from these services. It is therefore imperative that reablement is right for the individual at point of referral – that it is not used as a 'substitute' for a service that can-not be provided or, in the worst-case scenario, to make way for a vacant hospital bed.

Summary

➤ Reablement or restorative care in the UK, the USA, New Zealand and Australia requires a move from a culture of dependency and co-dependency between car-ers, people that use the service and statutory services, to adopting a more 'can-do' approach.

➤ Reablement services fall under the umbrella term of intermediate care.

➤ Intermediate care is a 'half-way home' service.

➤ The aim of reablement is to enable a person's autonomy at home, not just to maintain their current situation effectively.

➤ Broadly speaking, there are three types of reablement service model: hospital discharge; intake and assessment; and an integrated model. These all differ in process alongside agency involvement and team structure.

➤ Reablement may well be outsourced to home care agencies, but different access and attention to social activities, rather than just primary needs, would be the right move in the future.

Recommended reading

WILDE, A. & GLENDINNING, C. (2012) 'If they're helping me then how can I be independent?' The perceptions and experience of users of home-care re-ablement services. *Health and Social Care in the Community*, vol. 20, no. 6, 583–590.

▶

◄

E-learning resources

Useful for reablement support staff, professionals and managers alike

SCIE (SOCIAL CARE INSTITUTE FOR EXCELLENCE). (2013) *Reablement for care workers*. Available at: http://www.scie.org.uk/publications/elearning/reablement/ (Accessed 20 February 2015).
SCIE (SOCIAL CARE INSTITUTE FOR EXCELLENCE). (2013) *Reablement for managers*. Available at: http://www.scie.org.uk/assets/elearning/reablement/ module_1_web/index.html (Accessed 20 February 2015).

References

AGE UK. (2014) Loneliness in later life. Evidence review. Available at: http://www.ageuk.org.uk/Documents/EN-GB/For-professionals/Research/Evidence_Review-Loneliness_2014.pdf?dtrk=true (Accessed 12 June 2013).

BEAUMONT, J. (2013) Measuring national well-being – Older people and loneliness. Available at: http://webarchive.nationalarchives.gov.uk/20160105160709/http://www.ons.gov.uk/ons/dcp171766_304939.pdf. (Accessed 15 June 2017).

BERESFORD, P. (2015) *User involvement: Looking to the future*. Research in Practice for Adults (RiPFA). Available at: https://www.ripfa.org.uk/blog/user-involve-ment-looking-to-the-future/ (Accessed 12 January 2016).

CAMPAIGN TO END LONELINESS. (2011) *Loneliness research.* Available at: http://www.campaigntoendloneliness.org/loneliness-research/ (Accessed 20 February 2015).

COCHRANE, A. (2015) *Email Communication.* Discussion on unpublished results on a systematic review of reablement in marinating and improving older adult's functional independence.

COCHRANE, A., MCGILLOWAY, S., FURLONG, M., MOLLOY, D., STEVEN-SON, M. & DONNELLY, M. (2013) Home-care 'reablement' services for maintaining and improving older adults' functional independence. *The Cochrane Database of Systematic Reviews*, No. 11. DOI: 10.1002/14651858. CD010825.

COT (COLLEGE OF OCCUPATIONAL THERAPISTS). (2013) Reablement: The added value of occupational therapists. Available at: http://www.cot.co.uk/sites/default/files/position_statements/public/Position%20Statement%20Reablement.pdf (Accessed 20 April 2014).

CRANK, S. (2013) Conference, 2 October: Reablement away day, Cheshire West and Chester Council, Castle Park, Frodsham.

CSED (CARE SERVICES EFFICIENCY DELIVERY). (2007) *Homecare reablement workstream*, Discussion Document No. HRA 002, Department of Health, London.

CSED (CARE SERVICES EFFICIENCY DELIVERY). (2009) *Homecare Reablement, Prospective Longitudinal Study*, Interim Report 1 of 2. Department of Health, London.

CSED (CARE SERVICES EFFICIENCY DELIVERY). (2010a) Homecare re-ablement toolkit: What is homecare re-ablement? A definition. Available at: http://webarchive.nationalarchives.gov.uk/20120907090857/http://www.csed.dh.gov.uk/homeCareReablement/Toolkit/vision/#item2 (Accessed 28 October 2017).

CSED (CARE SERVICES EFFICIENCY DELIVERY). (2010b) Intermediate care and homecare re-ablement: What's in a name? Available at: http://webarchive.nationalarchives.gov.uk/20120907090129/http:/csed.dh.gov.uk/asset.cfm?aid=6647 (Accessed 28 October 2017).

Csikszentmihalyi, M. (1990). *Flow: The psychology of optimal experience*. Harper Perennial: New York

DAVIDSON, S. (2014) *Evidence review: Loneliness in later life*. Age UK. Available at: http://www.ageuk.org.uk/professional-resources-home/knowledge-hub-evidence-statistics/evidence-reviews/ (Accessed 7 September 2014).

DH (DEPARTMENT OF HEALTH). (2001) *National Service framework: Older people*. London: Department of Health. Available at: https://www.gov.uk/government/publications/quality-standards-for-care-services-for-older-people (Accessed 28 October 2017).

DH (DEPARTMENT OF HEALTH). (2002) *Intermediate care: Moving forward; National Service framework for older people supporting implementation*. London: Department of Health. Available at: http://webarchive.nationalarchives.gov.uk/+/http://www.dh.gov.uk/en/Publicationsandstatistics/Publications/PublicationsPolicyAndGuidance/DH_4006996?PageOperation=email (Accessed 28 October 2017).

DH (DEPARTMENT OF HEALTH). (2007a) *Homecare reablement workstream*. CSED. Discussion Document No. HRA 002, London: Department of Health.

DH (DEPARTMENT OF HEALTH). (2007b) *Putting people first: a shared vision and commitment to the transformation of adult social care*. Available at: http://webarchive.nationalarchives.gov.uk/20130107105354/http:/www.dh.gov.uk/en/Publicationsandstatistics/Publications/PublicationsPolicyAndGuidance/DH_081118 (Accessed 21 July 2016).

DH (DEPARTMENT OF HEALTH). (2010) *Prioritising need in the context of putting people first: A whole system approach to eligibility for social care*. London: Department of Health. Available at: http://webarchive.nationalarchives.gov.uk/20130105053920/http://www.dh.gov.uk/en/Publicationsandstatistics/Publications/PublicationsPolicyAndGuidance/DH_113154 (Accessed 29 October 2017).

DH (DEPARTMENT OF HEALTH). (2012) *Caring for our future: Reforming care and support*. London: The Stationery Office. Available at: https://www.gov.uk/government/publications/caring-for-our-future-reforming-care-and-support (Accessed 28 October 2017).

DH (DEPARTMENT OF HEALTH). (2014a) *Care Act 2014*. Available at: http://www.legislation.gov.uk/ukpga/2014/23/contents/enacted (Accessed 28 October 2017).

DH (DEPARTMENT OF HEALTH). (2014b) *Guidance: Care Act factsheets.* Updated April 2016. Available at: https://www.gov.uk/government/ publications/care-act-2014-part-1-factsheets/care-act-factsheets (Accessed 21 July 2016).

FOX, A., LOCKWOOD, S., STANSFIELD, J., WATERS, J., ELWELL, L. & BROAD, R. (2012) *Redesigning the front end of social care.* Available at: http://www. in-control.org.uk/media/113561/redesigning%20the%20front%20end%20 of%20social%20care%20final.pdf (Accessed 28 October 2017).

GERALD PILKINGTON ASSOCIATES. (2011) *The outsourcing of homecare re-ablement.* Available at: http://www.geraldpilkingtonassociates.com/js/ plugins/filemanager/files/OUTSOURCING_HOMECARE_RE-ABLEMENT_ SERVICES.pdf (Accessed 28 October 2017).

GLENDINNING, C. (2013) *Home care reablement services: Impacts and cost-effectiveness.* Plenary. Social Care 2013 Conference, London, 13 March.

GLENDINNING, C. & NEWBRONNER, E. (2008) The effectiveness of home care reablement – developing the evidence base 2008. *Journal of Integrated Care,* vol. 16, no. 4, 32–39.

HEALTH AND SOCIAL CARE BOARD. (2015) *Regional review of reablement services: Overview report.* Belfast: Health and Social Care Board. Available at: http://www.hscboard.hscni.net/board/meetings/May%202015/Item%20 16%20%2002%20-%20Regional%20Reablement%20overview%20report%20 PDF%20948KB.pdf (Accessed 20 November 2015).

INTERLINKS. (n.d.) *Home care re-ablement: Policy and Governance.* Available at: http://interlinks.euro.centre.org/model/example/HomeCareReAblement (Accessed 21 November 2014).

KENT, J., PAYNE, C., STEWART, M. & UNELL, J. (2000) *External evaluation of the Home Care Re-ablement Pilot Project.* Leicester: Centre for Group Care and Community Care Studies, De Montfort University.

MCGREGOR, K. (2013) *How one council is attempting to reduce demand on statutory social work services.* Community Care, 2 September. Available at: http://www.communitycare.co.uk/2013/09/02/how-one-council-is-attempting-to-reduce-demand-on-statutory-social-work-services/ (Accessed 28 October 2017).

MANTHORPE, J. (2011) *Long term impact of home care reablement.* Community Care, 13 October, 32–33. Available at: https://www.scie-socialcareonline.org. uk/long-term-impact-of-home-care-reablement/r/a1CG0000000GgLCMA0 (Accessed 28 October 2017).

MASI, C. M., CHEN, H.-Y., HAWKLEY, L. C. & CACIOPPO, J. M. (2011) A meta-analysis of interventions to reduce loneliness. *Personality and Social Psychology Review,* vol. 15, no. 3, 219–266.

MICKEL, A. (2010) Rethinking reablement. *Occupational Therapy News,* vol. 18, no. 11, 36–37.

MILLER, E. (2014) *Embedding outcomes in reablement in North Lanarkshire: Summary report.* Glasgow: University of Strathclyde. Available at: https:// personaloutcomes.files.wordpress.com/2014/03/summary-outcomes-in-reablement-report.pdf. (Accessed 15 January 2018).

NEIEP (NORTH EAST IMPROVEMENT AND EFFICIENCY PARTNERSHIP).
(2010) *Reablement: A guide for frontline staff*. London: Office for Public
Management.

NEWTON, C. (2012) Personalising reablement: Inserting the missing link.
Working with Older People, vol. 16, no. 3, 117–121.

NICE (NATIONAL INSTITUTE FOR CLINICAL EXCELLENCE). (2013) *Falls:
Assessment and prevention of falls in older people. Clinical guideline 161*, London:
NICE.

PILKINGTON, G. (2008) Homecare re-ablement: Why and how providers and
commissioners can implement a service. *Journal of Care Services Management*,
vol. 2, no. 4, 354–367.

PITTS, J., SANDERSON, H., WEBSTER, A. & SKELLHORN, L. (2011) *A new
reablement journey*. Available at: https://www.choiceforum.org/docs/rea.pdf
(Accessed 28 October 2017).

RABIEE, P. & GLENDINNING, C. (2011) Organisation and delivery of homecare
reablement: what makes a difference? *Health and Social Care in the Community*, vol. 19, no. 5, 495–503.

REGAN, B., WELLS, Y. & FOREMAN, P. (2009) Enabling independence: Restorative approaches to home care provision for frail older adults. *Health and
Social Care in the Community*, vol. 17, no. 3, 225–234.

ROBB, B. (2013) Why social workers want to help redesign homecare services.
The Guardian, 15 November.

SAMUEL, M. (2012) Reablement success leads to social work job cuts. *Community Care*, 22 February.

SANDERSON, H. & LEWIS, J. (2012) *A practical guide to delivering personalisation:
Person centred practice in health and social care*. London: Jessica Kingsley.

SCIE (SOCIAL CARE INSTITUTE FOR EXCELLENCE). (2011a) *Reablement:
Emerging practice messages*. Available at: http://www.scie.org.uk/files/
EmergingMessages.pdf (Accessed 15 January 2018).

SCIE (SOCIAL CARE INSTITUTE FOR EXCELLENCE). (2011b) *Briefing 36. Reablement: A cost-effective route to better outcomes*. Available at: http://www.scie.org.
uk/publications/briefings/briefing36 (Accessed 15 January 2018).

SCIE (SOCIAL CARE INSTITUTE FOR EXCELLENCE). (2012a) *Guide 47: Personalisation: A rough guide*. London: SCIE.

SCIE (SOCIAL CARE INSTITUTE FOR EXCELLENCE). (2012b) *At a glance 56:
Making the move to delivering reablement*. Available at: https://www.scie.org.
uk/publications/ataglance/ataglance56.asp (Accessed 8 January 2015).

SCIE (SOCIAL CARE INSTITUTE FOR EXCELLENCE). (2012c) *At a glance 52:
reablement: Key issues for commissioners of adult social care*. London: SCIE.

SCIE (SOCIAL CARE INSTITUTE FOR EXCELLENCE). (2013) *Fair access to care
services (FACS): Prioritising eligibility for care and support*. Available at: http://
www.scie.org.uk/publications/guides/guide33/files/guide33.pdf (Accessed
12 January 2015).

SCIE (SOCIAL CARE INSITUTE FOR EXCELLENCE). (2015) *Care Act 2014:
Assessment and eligibility process map*. Available at: http://www.scie.org.uk/care-
act-2014/assessment-and-eligibility/process-map/ (Accessed 12 January 2015).

SKELTON, J. (2013) Why occupational therapists are central to Reablement services. *The Guardian*, 25 October.

THE ATKINSON. (2014) *The Atkinson Festival of Wellbeing: Getting the most out of life*. Available at: http://www.ageconcernliverpoolandsefton.org.uk/wp-content/uploads/2014/09/Festival-of-Wellbeing-brochure.pdf (Accessed 12 November 2014).

THINK LOCAL ACT PERSONAL. (2011) *Personal budgets: Taking stock, moving forward*. Available at: http://www.thinklocalactpersonal.org.uk/

U3A. (2014) The Westerly: News blowing in from Westerham U3A. Available at: http://www.westerhamu3a.org/uploads/7/2/4/0/7240242/the_westerly_1.pdf (Accessed 28 October 2017).

VICTOR, C., BOWLING, A., SCAMBLER, S. & BOND, J. (2003) *Loneliness, social isolation and living alone in later life*. Sheffield: ESRC Growing Older Programme.

WILDE, A. & GLENDINNING, C. (2012) 'If they're helping me then how can I be independent?' The perceptions and experience of users of home-care reablement services. *Health & Social Care in the Community*, vol. 20, no. 6, 583–590.

WOOD, C. & SALTER, J. (2012) *The home cure*. London: Demos. Available at: http://www.demos.co.uk/files/Home_Cure_-_web_1_.pdf?1340633545 (Accessed 15 January 2018).

4

Undoing Dependence: Promoting Autonomy

V. Ebrahimi and S. Phillips

Chapter outline

It has long been recognised that health care, in essence, is paternalistic. This approach to practice instils a dependency relationship between service provider and the 'end user' (Thompson 2012). Much the same can be said about social care despite the 'affiliation' by many to a **social model (disability)** of practice. Historically, the public understanding of this dependency relationship can (often) be summed up through the use of metaphors that infantilise older people, for example as being *'warm and incompetent'*. Furthermore, and as Thompson (2011) argues, the infantilising language by professionals (baby talk and patronising), although sometimes a deliberate 'put down', is more often used without thought and is an 'unwitting' misuse of power. This way of being was argued by Hockey and James as the 'manifestations of a key logical cognitive structure through which human dependency is created and re-created in Western cultures' (Hockey and James 1993, cited in Thompson 2011, p. 95). It is argued here that this ideology continues in the way in which broader society in the UK perceives the older person. Despite the advent of health promotion in the early part of the twenty-first century and public health initiatives, the metaphors and language of health professionals in the UK remain similar to that described by Thompson (2011).

Being alone, as indicated in reviews of evidence by Age UK (2014), means that dependence on another for food, shelter and security increases for some. From a threat-to-survival position this prompts individuals to do something about it – thus ensuring survival. This dynamic changes, however, when loneliness becomes chronic, affecting health and well-being. The implications of loneliness for some is that their needs may go unnoticed so that by the time they are known to a service their health has often deteriorated significantly. Most often in the discharge of older people from hospital a dependency relationship is fostered through formal care. This can also be seen in instances where there has been a breakdown in communication or ineffective co-ordination (co-working) among community services. Despite meeting the daily living needs of millions of people, formal care is often seen as a way out for some, in their attempt to combat loneliness and so the cycle is perpetuated. This is therefore a false **dichotomy**. We meet the daily living needs of the person, as well as providing some 'social contact' (ironically), but purposefully, or out of ignorance, ignore other more useful alternatives. The health and social care system, as it stands in the current climate, needs to start 'undoing' these dependency relationships with thoughtfulness, while still addressing the genuine need for paid care when and if it arises.

Throughout this book we argue that reablement is not about being tied to a specific location (the person's home), but is rather a way of being (interacting) – an ethos. It is therefore critical that there is understanding of how dependence manifests which, for several older adults, leads to situations of learned helplessness, aided by the maintenance of dependent relationships. The inherent nature of reablement is to move away from the notion (or assumption) of 'incompetence' or lack of ability to one which is open to **self-determination**. We have a concerted duty to promote autonomy – not just for ourselves for the future but because we cannot continue with this kind of dependence due to the implications this has on the economy. This idea is reflected in the early Department of Health (DH 2007) concordat which sought to put 'People First' through radical reform and transformation in adult social care. It is also manifest in many other legislative contexts.

Chapter objectives

By the end of this chapter you should be able to:

➢ Discuss a range of definitions and perceptions of independence (autonomy)

➢ Consider factors that may enhance or detract from establishing personalised autonomy

➢ Examine how specific models of care and ideologies may work for or against the reforms promoting 'independent or autonomous living'[1]

➢ Assess how reablement can change society's perceptions of ability in older adults living at home alongside those of their informal carers

---

[1] It is worth noting here that there are many references to key authors from the 1990s. This is deliberate as many of the ideas discussed relate to seminal work and therefore this requires acknowledgement.

What is the meaning of 'independence'?

At first sight, independence is a concept that lends itself to a common-sense interpretation – that of not relying on other people for one's needs. However, this requires further exploration in the context of reablement. Although the philosophy of reablement is to promote independence and avoid creating dependence, **definitions of 'independence'** will vary from person to person, and indeed between different service providers. To support workers and professionals, a person may be deemed to be 'independent' when they can manage general activities of daily living (ADL). Let's look at this in a bit more detail.

Typically, reablement programmes focus on dressing, walking up and down stairs, washing, and preparing meals (Francis, Fisher and Rutter 2011), and evaluations of the effectiveness of reablement interventions again are centred on the need for further physical care (Lewin et al. 2013). However, this may limit a person's independence meaning that other areas of life are neglected. There may be conflict between different expectations of independence – for example, social engagement, where service users may welcome the social interaction with support workers (Wilde and Glendinning 2012) as opposed to the difficulties associated with getting out/leaving the home for this purpose. So reablement may only enable one aspect of what people understand as independence: being more physically able. One service user comments after a reablement intervention that: *'[I] got a bit stronger maybe, but it didn't do anything [for me] mentally'* (Trappes-Lomax and Hawton 2012, p. 186). Here a physical outcome is recognised but the participant in this study finds something is lacking. We could perhaps suggest this to be meaningful social contact or purposeful activity. There are other outcomes, however, that should also be considered, namely changes in the individual's life, for example perceived quality of life and well-being (Francis, Fisher and Rutter 2011). Importantly this factor may have a profound influence on whether an individual maintains his or her level of independence following reablement.

Conceptual definitions of dependence and independence

Concepts of dependence and independence in a health care context are often shaped by professional thinking and practice (Goble 2014). The general pattern of professional intervention, including decision making, follows a linear process on initial contact with the person:

Assessment → **Clinical reasoning** → **Intervention** → **Evaluation**

An assessment enables identification of issues or difficulties (physical, cognitive, emotional), which leads to the professional determining what development and subsequent intervention are required, including equipment, aids and adaptations. For example, a person recovering from a stroke needs to be taught new techniques through facilitation to enable them to wash themselves. Despite the obvious benefit of this, there are nonetheless contentions. Even if there is an emphasis on 'person-centred care', there may be pressure on the individual to conform to a passive 'sick role', to go along with the programme or intervention, and to accept the expert verdict on its effectiveness. There may even be a subtle pressure to be grateful for this caring attention and to be as little bother as possible to the busy 'caring professional'. As Goble (2014, p. 33) suggests, 'Stepping outside the parameters of this role is to risk being characterised as ungrateful or difficult'. It may be particularly challenging for people with intellectual or vocal impairment to articulate their needs and opinions. This is revisited later (see the section 'Service land') in the example of a woman with learning difficulties reliant on a wheelchair and regular support from a formal carer. Being dependent on carers (whether paid or not) may also initiate and sustain social contact, and therefore service users may be reluctant to sever this relationship. Acknowledgement of this, offering mutually agreed alternatives, may be helpful in these instances. Consider Scenario 4.1 in the facilitation of independence for a person we have called Beth. See if you can make suggestions on how to motivate her and enable her to be more autonomous.

Scenario 4.1   Facilitation of autonomy: Beth

Beth is 78 years old and had a **subarachnoid haemorrhage** approximately two years ago. Aside from some difficulties with walking, Beth is relatively independent. The greatest impact of the stroke, however, is in the limitation of being able to raise her hands and arms any further upwards than her chest. This complicates matters for her with all sorts of ADL (person, domestic and social) and up until now she has had formal care input every morning. A decision was made with Beth to try reablement for three weeks and review this at week four. Every morning your aim is to encourage her to wash her face and brush her teeth. You can tell, however, that she is often uncomfortable and often frowns so you try to offer alternatives. In response Beth often just says 'I couldn't manage without you … you are very kind. Thank you.'

Thursday morning week two

Q. Is Beth's response assertive or passive?

Q. What kind of indicators can you pick up from Beth's usual response to your questions?

Q. Is there something else you could do to help motivate her and improve the situation?

For the most part in health and social care services, there is a risk of assuming 'any standard' or 'simple concept' of independence in the delivery of reablement interventions. Meanings of independence are multifaceted, personal and subject to change as individuals' circumstances change (Wilde and Glendinning 2012). Indeed, and in the instance of long-term conditions (LTCs), as will be discussed in Chapter 6, a person's health is never linear but is better described as dynamic – shifting and changing with time. Added to this may be a tension between the inherent aims of reablement and pressure to reduce cost of care (either paid or unpaid services). There may also be a tension between 'costs' – for example, the drive for 'independence' or autonomy, when a person is deemed to be no longer in need of care and support – and the actual 'wants' of service users. Equally there may also be conflict in the way carers (both formal and informal) behave towards the service users – for example, between 'doing for' and 'letting do'. This will be explored further in the next chapter when discussing the training and education of support workers and/or formal carers.

Society often has expectations of what people with disabilities and impairment can do – for example, what is 'normal' (Cameron 2014) – and there is a clear need for discussion and negotiation so that boundaries, both real and perceived, are identified. This perspective is also seen in many of the examples of working with older people with limiting physical ability or conditions. Some may be in denial of impairment, which can subsequently limit the journey to autonomy. These individuals will need help to come to terms with the associated difficulties, without becoming depressed, uncertain of their future and hence demotivated. Some people will have unrealistic expectations of their ability or potential. This could be either because of a mental health difficulty, cognitive capacity or insight (into one's own situation or health) or because of another health-related 'problem'. An example of this might be in the instance of impaired **neuropsychological processing**. Assessment may be needed in this instance to determine the involvement of brain injury following trauma or a neurological illness. Despite all this we can still work in partnership with care and thought with an aim to instil trust in our actions as professionals and support staff. What may be perceived as insurmountable may actually not be too far off. So perhaps there is just a greater need to demonstrate patience, to offer more time (or a skilled semblance of it) and, importantly, even if we cannot truly understand individual experience, we can still show our appreciation when a person 'dares to share'.

Pre-existing conditions may preclude some independence in ADL, as with certain mental health or progressive conditions (Wilde and Glendinning 2012) such as dementia. Equally, the environment may predispose to dependence or independence. For example, Trappes-Lomax and Hawton's (2012) research explored older people's experiences of reablement and rehabilitation, and found hospital routines may enforce dependence: 'you do get very dependent in hospital, someone tells you when it's time to do things and what to do and where to go' (p. 187). Whereas in the same study, people welcomed the chance of 'doing it for yourself' (p. 186) in rehabilitation settings. Disability writers address the concepts of 'independence' and 'autonomy' from yet another perspective. Fine and Glendinning (2005) illustrate this perspective well by suggesting that independence needs to be understood not as being able to perform activities for oneself without help, but as being able to exercise control over what help is needed. Here perhaps is also a distinction between being able to make decisions for oneself and perhaps needing help in carrying out the results of those decisions. This requires a different mindset for carers working with service users, both informal carers and health and social care professionals. It is about being facilitative and person-centred, rather than directive and 'overly' active. Let's now look at this in the context of Beth who we considered earlier in Scenario 4.1.

Student Activity 4.1   Encouraging motivation: Connecting with Beth

---

Looking back at Scenario 4.1 Beth agreed to reablement so that she could have more autonomy in washing her face and therefore be less reliant on formal care. Nonetheless, she clearly lacks motivation as the weeks progress. Do you think Beth has a sense of purpose during the interventions and is she in control? Have a look at the following suggestions and statements:

Have a collection of easy-read articles in your office/car:

'Beth, look at this article I found for you [**personalise it**]. *It talks about how being more in control of your own personal care can have benefits in lots of ways!'*

'I don't know what it is like to have to relearn to wash your face [**connection and understanding**], *but I thought the article was really interesting. What do you think?'*

'Hmm ... we have tried to do it this way using a long-reach handle but I recently saw how to adapt one with a sponge by sticking some Velcro to it ... Shall we have a go? [**suggesting alternatives and working in partnership**].

'It will probably feel a bit awkward at first but it might work for you' [**acknowledgement and support**].

To enable someone to have more control they need to be less passive and more active. You may find that different approaches work at different times, depending on the person's mood, culture and spiritual beliefs, so be flexible. But(!) always work in

▶

◄

partnership. Make the person feel that it is a partnership and that whatever the intervention it coexists with equal effort.

Some days the person will struggle, but always find something positive to say and
ignore any negativity. Respond to statements like *'I couldn't manage without you ...
you are very kind. Thank you.'* with *'Oh but you managed without me! You are washing your face by yourself – isn't that right?'* **(positive reinforcement)**.

Some service users may demand a fair amount of time in helping to
regain their autonomy, and this can be particularly difficult when family or friends were previously involved in care. This means that the time
taken to achieve a task or even make a decision may be a very important
factor in allowing control to remain with the service user.

Dependency and interdependency

Definitions of care and carer are open to debate, particularly, as just discussed, when family or spouses are involved in care. Corden and Hirst
(2011) discuss instances of reciprocal care, which challenges formal
distinctions between care giver and care receiver. Part of their research
involved interviews with couples involved in end-of-life care for their
partner. Even in this extreme situation, more than one in ten reported
receiving care from the partner who died – the prevalence did not diminish as the partners approached death. Four per cent of couples could be
described as mutual care givers at the interview before a death, and in 7%
of cases only the partner who died was described as providing care.

Reflection Point 4.1   Caring for a 'dependant' and the mirror of
frustration

Standing back and watching your partner or relative struggle with everyday tasks is
difficult. Not only does it raise feelings such as anger, guilt, pity and impatience, but
also the sense that by not helping it is unkind. The impact of this is that we treat
people differently but also in a very obvious way. The more we do this, the more the
recipient feels the same: guilt, anger and often immense frustration. Relationships
then become difficult as each day is fraught with tension alongside the enduring
physical and emotive demands of both recipient and care giver/s. This can be likened
to a mirror of frustration because it occurs at the same time and is perceived simulta-
neously by both care giver and receiver.

Goble (2014) explores the links between dependence and inter-dependence, concluding that: 'we are all who we are because of our interrelationship with others, and we are all "independent" because we are inter-dependent' (p. 36). This paints the concept of 'dependency' in a different light, perhaps suggesting that it is a professionally defined issue that has little relevance in 'real life', and may in fact perpetuate the idea of the 'sick role'.

The sick role

Parsons (1951, cited in Barnes 2014) viewed 'sickness', both short and long term, as a deviation from the 'normal' state of being, and people who are sick have certain rights, for example, being relieved of their usual roles and responsibilities. As Goble (2014) points out, this may lead to an expectation by care professionals that the disabled person will conform to this role and go along with prescribed programmes or interventions. However, Parsons has been criticised for, among other things, the inapplicability of the sick role to chronic illness, and indeed, whether being ill or disabled is, in fact, socially deviant. In a modern context, service users are encouraged to take on a non-passive role in acceptance of their own care, to question their treatment and to 'shop-around' for the best care (Williams 2005), which may in itself add to the vulnerability and confusion of frail elderly people. Parsons talks about the 'inequality' in the doctor–patient relationship, where the doctor is seen as the expert and the patient as the lay person who will accept the doctor's superior knowledge and guidance. This may be translated into today's multidisciplinary team perhaps, but the relationship may still be considered as unequal according to Parsons' criteria, even taking into account increased lay knowledge and 'expert patient' criteria (Lupton 1996, cited in Williams 2005). Such relationships are ideally based upon trust and **rapport** between the carer and the cared-for. This then opens further the debate on the concepts discussed in Chapter 2 about person-centred care and what is meant by this term. Let's appraise this further.

Person-centred care

Person-centred care was one of the principles set out in the National Service Framework for Older People, a ten-year programme for improving services for this group with a series of reviews five and seven years later (DH 2001; Commission for Healthcare Audit and Inspection 2006; Darzi 2008). The concept of a person-centred approach seems to lack an agreed definition, but a common theme arising involves individualisation of health care interventions and shared decision making and goal set-ting, as defined by Schmitt, Akroyd and Burke (2012). Their research with physiotherapy students on perceptions of person-centred care resembles those perceptions defined by health care professionals, while those of service users differed. In particular, co-ordination and smooth transition between services was seen as important by service users, but little men-tioned by the physiotherapy students. Similarly, the concept of patient empowerment was important to the students, whereas service users did not see this in the same way. If it is the case that the understanding of the concept differs perhaps Nolan and colleagues (2004), undertaking research into nursing practice, have a valid argument that person-centred care may perpetuate poor standards of care for older people, rather than eliminate them. They suggest that the vision of person-centred care is 'contemporary speak' which is untenable in the context of health care for older people, and instead suggest 'relationship-centred care', includ-ing valuing interdependence and the contribution of family and others who support a disabled person. Hebblethwaite's (2013) research supports this, stating: 'both terms are given prominence in mission and philoso-phy statements, but found tensions exist when these are implemented in practice' (p. 13). Her work with therapeutic recreation specialists found that although the practitioners subscribed to the concepts, and often made a point of changing practice to try to facilitate service users' wishes, they were constrained by issues such as scheduling of meals and the chal-lenges of interdisciplinary teamwork, for example. One theme found was that one of the biggest barriers to implementing patient-centred care was the emphasis on loss, dependency and impairment found in some profes-sional groups, rather than a focus on people's strengths and abilities.

What helps and what hinders

The primary aim of reablement is to change the philosophy from one where delivery of care may create dependency to provision of care which maximises independence, self-esteem and health-related quality of life (HRQoL), thereby reducing care input (Parsons et al. 2012). Parsons and colleagues (2012) conclude that key elements in creating independence are goal facilitation, functional and repetitive exercises to improve mobil-ity and activity, support worker training and enhanced supervision, and health professional training and care management. Reablement should not be a catch-all service. Some people may still require formal care, for example with assistance in morning dressing as a result of daily exacerba-tion of rheumatoid arthritis, often more acutely felt on rising.

Rabiee and Glendinning's (2011) qualitative study explores which factors in the organisation, delivery and content of reablement services have the potential to enhance or detract from their effectiveness. Key points arising from this study were that reablement seems to have more benefits for people recovering from falls and acute illnesses, rather than more chronic conditions or multiple impairments. On the other hand, there are few if any other studies to date to compare this with. Second, clear outcomes for users (or goal setting) were found to be a requirement, together with the flexibility to adapt these as needs change. Third, Rabiee and Glendinning (2011) concur that wider environmental success factors include shared vision between people and carers, and access to specialist support and adequate capacity in long-term home care. Co-production is an example of genuine partnership. This was discussed in Chapter 2 and the theme continues in subsequent chapters. From another competing perspective and in order to gradually make changes to the traditional output of paid care, it is important to understand the impact of the notion of 'service land' on recipients. To understand the complexities of this it is useful to take a few steps back and consider discourse – in particular dominant and countervailing ideologies. This is now explained in more detail.

The medical model and service land

Dominant ideologies

Discourse relates to the way in which language is used to shape sets of meanings used to think, understand and communicate. Medical discourse is explained by Saraga (1998) as a system that frames disability as a condition of 'biophysical essence' and origin. Individuals are seen as unable to perform expected, valued and typical human activities as a consequence of impairment and disability. This type of health discourse has a close relationship with power and helps to maintain the oppression of people with disabilities. Thompson (1998, p. 137) illustrates this idea well in his representation of medical discourse and the status quo (see Figure 4.1).

Although Thompson (1998) explains the relationship and influence of language on oppression in terms of 'the medical profession', this is not confined only to doctors and nurses, but to a whole array of both health and social care professions, as well as those in the private sector (for example, nursing, residential and care homes). In the instance of reablement we must be aware of this. Despite the argument by some that there is more of an alliance with a social model (explained below), because of reablement's location in communities (people's homes) there are instances where patronising language is in use. One example is the term 'compliance', sometimes used when a person does not conform to

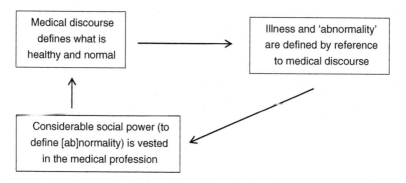

Figure 4.1   Medical discourse and the status quo
Source: Thompson (1998)

the use of suggested equipment, method of transfer or medication. It goes without saying that people with LTCs must have, and will always need, support from services in health and social care. What is obvious, however, from Figure 4.1 is the process in which the dominant ideology – of what is normal and what is not (subtle) – is maintained by the medical establishment. Medical discourse thus creates the potential, as Thompson (1998, p. 69) states, for 'powerful people to present their own construction of the world'. This effectively protects and consolidates positions of power at the expense of the less powerful: people with disabilities, impairments or chronic conditions who rely on outsider help. This is even more so in the case in services where the majority of users are older people and in instances where they have short- or long-term mental health issues, memory loss or learning difficulties.

The medical model (or the notions associated with it) therefore has and continues to have a significant impact on the way in which services are delivered. The ideas associated with this were noted as far back as the 1990s by Thompson (1998), Barnes, Mercer and Shakespeare (1999) and Marks (1999). Moreover, its major influence – we will state here for argument's sake – is, to some extent, the restriction of people's right to lead autonomous lives, characterised by choice. The close alignment between medicine and occupational therapy (OT), for instance, was evident to Sumsion and Smyth (2000) and Turner (1997) who described them as 'uneasy bedfellows'. This tension is experienced by many an OT and continues today within a profession that was at one time known as 'supplementary to medicine'. It is now, however, more than ever, that OT may really come into its own and be more clearly understood by commissioners and the public alike. This is argued as another discourse that merits far wider discussion elsewhere. You may recall the ideas associated with mindfulness and person-centred practice, in relation to occupations that include control, meaning and choice (Chapter 2). It makes sense then at this juncture to look at this facet of health service provision in relation to the opposite to medical models of care.

Countervailing ideologies

So far as dominant ideologies exist, such as the medical model, so do oppositional countervailing ones. For example, activists in the disability movement support a countervailing ideology. Their main argument against several dominant ideologies and discourses is that it is the social order, including services, that must change, not people with disabilities (Thompson 1998; Kendrick 2000). The social model of disability sees the experience of disability not as an effect of impairment, but caused by the relationship between the individual and their environmental barriers (Barton and Oliver 1997; Marks 1999). The use of technology to support people in their home and social environments is given closer scrutiny in Chapter 8. In the UK, the social model of disability arose as a result of a seminal publication in 1976 produced by the Union of the Physically Impaired Against Segregation (UPIAS) and the Disability Alliance. The statement given in Box 4.1 sums up very adequately this ideology, which, in a contemporary context, can perhaps now be more accurately understood as the social/political model of disability.

Box 4.1   Declaration of the fundamental principles of disability

A tape-recorded discussion between the Disability Alliance and the UPIAS:

disability is a situation, caused by social conditions, which requires for its elimination, (a) that no one aspect such as incomes, mobility or institutions is treated in isolation, (b) that disabled people should, with the advice and help of others, assume control over their own lives, and (c) that professionals, experts and others who seek to help must be committed to promoting such control by disabled people.

(UPIAS and the Disability Alliance 1975, p. 3)

Given the above declaration can we state with conviction that the move to give more control to service users, more than 40 years later, is evident? To some extent yes, but clearly there is a way to go yet. Direct payments are one such move towards autonomy and this aspect is taken further shortly. Reablement is another. Essentially, however, service user groups and disability social theorists have argued that levels of independence (or autonomy) should relate to the control people have over their lives, rather than their ability to perform particular technical activities (Marks 1999; In Control 2014). This might mean that being able to drink a pint in a pub has more importance to an individual than whether they can tie their shoelaces or not.

Service land

There are criticisms of the medical and social model ideologies but these will not be explored any further here. What we can take from this, however, is that the social model helps us to recognise that health and social care services – among other societal influences – impact on people's choices and do create dependence. Historically, they have often served to a greater extent to empower service providers, much less the people that use the associated services. This may change in the current political climate as individuals gain greater control and say through social media.

Let us consider the dynamic of service land in relation to who the individual might come across in their journey through health and social care. The perspective of a person who needs to use a wheelchair helps to illustrate this dynamic. Once you have considered the content of the Box in 4.1, look at the illustration in Figure 4.2. This content is adapted from Munro and Elder-Woodward (1992) to reflect contemporary services today.

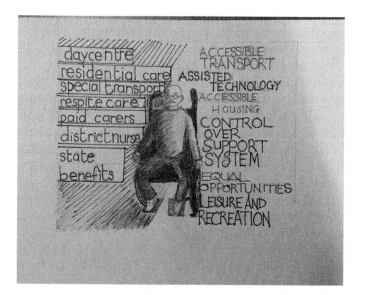

Figure 4.2   The contrast between service land and the ideology of choice and control

Source: Illustration by W. Chapman (2017)

What kind of differences do you think there are today in a person's health and social care journey compared to that of the early 1990s? Write your thoughts in Reflection Point 4.2:

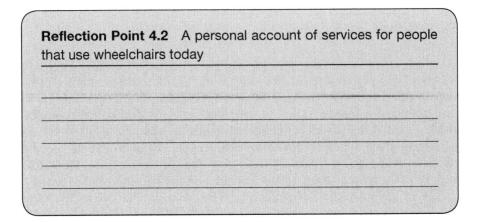

Reflection Point 4.2   A personal account of services for people that use wheelchairs today

Disability activists have always been strong advocates of providing a range of choices to service users, with the assertion that independence is equivalent to quality of life – *'with help'*. In Figure 4.2 the individual is empowered and has control of support systems either as a result of articulating their own goals (which could be leisure-related) or via an advocate such as a personal assistant (personal budget recipient). This facilitation towards empowerment can be seen to the right of the image. Aspects to the left show instances where control is lessened by services (disempowerment). Some people will want to have formal care assistance with all DADL except for meal preparation. Many older people dislike ready meals but this may be the only choice when being assisted by formal carers. Assistance might include acceptance (or not) of assistive technology such as telehealth or telecare (see Chapter 8) as well as adaptations (through-floor lift or level-access shower) and aids for daily living (jar-lid turner or pick-up stick) in their home. These all help support the person but ultimately should be in place through choice. At the same time, however, the individual is reliant on the professional telling them what is available and how long it might take. This should be done with accuracy, clarity and without undertone in relation to what the person should expect.

To add to the previous debate, it is worth thinking about how professionals, support workers and all those that work in the health and social care industry are equally reliant on individuals that need their expertise and care. Without them we would not exist, we would have no reason to get up in the morning; we would not get paid. To this extent, it is good to step back a bit and remember this. We need to 'just be' with the person whatever we choose to call him or her – service user, client, patient.

The oft-argued sentiment of trying to imagine what it is like to be in some-one else's situation, 'to crawl under their skin', is a rather **defunct** one. We can never understand this, or how people feel about relying (often heavily) on public services to be able to live a reasonable quality of life.

The reason then why it is important to understand these dynamics in the context of reablement is because dominant ideologies do nega-tively impact on older people with a disability, long-term condition or impairment. Indeed, you or your family may at some point require support from the array of health and social care services. You may also become an 'unwilling participant' as in the example taken below from an interview carried out in a undergraduate research study in Edinburgh, 2002:

> I wanted people to support me, not just do and take charge.

The above statement seems fairly self-explanatory until placed in the wider picture and context in which it was said. Patricia (pseudonym) had been asked what kind of qualities she would like in her staff (formal car-ers) and to provide a score between one and ten during a **Person-Centred Planning** (PCP) meeting. She described some attributes that she felt were important to her and these were then matched to her support staff. Patricia was in her early 70s, she had mild learning difficulties, used a wheelchair to get from one place to the next and required a significant amount of hands-on support with PADL (manual handling). It became apparent, however, during the PCP meeting that Patricia's key worker for nine years had a very low score (one). She described her as patronis-ing, abrupt and a person who did not listen to her – essentially uncaring. Following Patricia's revelation in the PCP meeting, she said during our interview that she 'burst into tears cos I had so much tension'. Patricia said that she had not realised how negatively her key worker had made her feel. She described feeling a lot of relief after this disclosure and subsequently it is understood that this formal carer was replaced with a **personal assistant**. This was based on active co-production which was discussed earlier in Chapter 2 (see the section 'Forwards to co-produc-tion') as well as feelings of helplessness in Chapter 7 which argues the theoretical basis for this in more depth. What we can take from Patricia's story is an understanding of how relationships between an individual and a formal carer can be very unequal – lacking in **choice, control** and **autonomy**. The reverse of this example is therefore **empowerment**.

In summary, we can see that oppression can be enforced through sev-eral means. This may be via political or clinical decision making, such as rights to timely surgical procedures, through monetary means, such as entitlement to state benefits, or when formal care is provided thought-lessly. The next example resonates more with how reablement can make very positive changes in dominant ideologies of formal care provision. It can help to change the ethos/philosophy of care provision as discussed earlier: 'service land'. An awareness, however, is critical in terms of how older adults from a wide range of different socio-economic circumstances perceive independence and what they consider important. So the next more current case example from Liverpool illustrates this, but first consider the statement in Reflection Point 4.3.

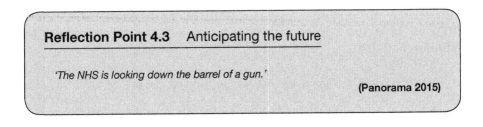

Reflection Point 4.3   Anticipating the future

'The NHS is looking down the barrel of a gun.'

(Panorama 2015)

Change practice, change lives

Liverpool is situated in the north-west of England and is known as the most health-deprived city in England. This problem is so serious that a task force involving hospital, local authority and voluntary service providers and experts has been drawn together with a particular focus and vision. The aim of the 'The Healthy Liverpool Programme' (LCCG 2015) is to find solutions to the overstretched NHS. Moving care to the community has been a driver for at least ten years but the *Panorama* programme reports that in only 24 months the NHS will grind to a halt. The plan therefore is city-wide engagement and tangible moves towards integrated care, including a timeline with an emphasis on health care in three settings, one of them named 'Living Well'. Supporting people to self-care and to make better and healthier lifestyle choices is the aim, with two out of the six priority areas focusing on healthy ageing and long-term conditions. For LTCs the ambition includes reducing:

➢ Coronary heart disease emergency admissions by 18.3% by 2018/19

➢ Emergency admissions for chronic obstructive pulmonary disease by 26.9% by 2018/19

➢ Potential years of life lost by 24.2% by 2018/19

For healthy ageing the aim of the programme is to increase the proportion of people still at home 90 days after hospital discharge and reduce permanent admissions for over 65s to residential and nursing homes.

Reducing emergency admissions for vertebral and hip fractures by a quarter is another ambitious target. What, however, should we all make of the following striking message stated in the programme:

> The reason why you are not feeling great is nothing medical ... It is more social and it is more about life itself than being depressed and needing drugs.
>
> (Panorama 2015)

Perhaps the questions in Reflection Point 4.4 make us feel uncomfortable, but so they should. Undeniably many older community dwellers seek comfort in daily visits, argued by many as providing valuable social contact. On the other hand, being able to go out to meet with others with similar interests is 'what we do' throughout life. The quality of relationships is certainly questionable when the person is paid to interact socially. Think about the questions in Reflection Point 4.4 and answer them honestly.

Reflection Point 4.4   The impact of providing unnecessary support

Does this person 'actually need' someone to visit them twice a day to get their breakfast and lunch?

Think about who is paying for this – the individual or the state?

If there is even a remote possibility that they could do these activities autonomously, is this level of intervention right?

Making your own breakfast and lunch may prevent deterioration in ability, health and well-being long term – **True or false?**

Making your own breakfast and lunch means that additional funds could be used to support/provide for something else – **True or false?**

How easy is it to enable service users to think differently about their potential and communicate this effectively and with conviction?

The role of communication in effecting reablement interventions

Explicit in the literature is the need to be overt with the service user and their family about the purpose of reablement, which is to minimise long-term care (Trappes-Lomax and Hawton 2012). The key to effective reablement appears in the way staff motivate people to engage. The experience of service users with reablement seems to be associated with the quality of the relationship they develop with their care workers, and, of course, communication is central to this. Wilde and Glendinning's (2012) research into service users' and carers' views of reablement highlighted that information was sometimes unavailable or inaccessible, was inappropriate to their situation or needs, or was given at an inappropriate time so that they were unable to make use it, or did not remember it. Wilde and Glendinning (2012) identify that service users' and (informal) carers' expectations were sometimes inappropriate, and that there was sometimes a lack of understanding of the aims of reablement. They also suggest that there may be conflict between expectations of independence. For example, some service users felt that reablement should include resuming social activities before other preliminary steps were taken – such as balance, stamina and overall safety when walking. Clear and timely communication is paramount and reablement teams must manage people's expectations from the outset, explaining not only the specific ethos of reablement, but also its boundaries in terms of the nature and length of support (Francis, Fisher and Rutter 2011). This may be particularly relevant for people who live alone, who may need careful and repeated information about the goals of reablement. Equally important is to establish service users' and carers' priorities in terms of what they hope to achieve. This must therefore involve setting short- and long-term goals for the duration of the six weeks.

The role of goal setting in effecting reablement interventions

It is suggested that realistic and relevant life goals should be negotiated jointly between service users and carers, and the skill of the therapist is crucial in determining these (Barnard, Cruice and Playford 2010, cited in Trappes-Lomax and Hawton 2012). This is in contrast to some who consider that the discussion on goal setting does not necessarily require a therapist. Many would argue, however, that those with appropriate training and education (OTs, PTs and experienced rehab nurses) are in a stronger position to determine if some goals are unrealistic, therefore averting individual 'failure'. This aspect of reablement merits further research.

Wilde and Glendinning (2012) identified some further constraints of goal setting. Some service users did not remember being involved in early goal setting, and therefore were unable to respond in relation to the achievement of these. Those who did recall the goals did, however, respond well. Again, this identifies the need for clear and repeated communication, particularly for those with newly diagnosed or progressive conditions, or a recent permanent impairment or disability. Service users who fail to make progress towards agreed goals risk becoming demoralised and this would be counterproductive. Thus goal setting not only needs to be articulated clearly and explicitly, but also requires skilled management, and careful and appropriate training of care workers. Importantly it is essential that goals are set in real partnerships.

FACT 4.1

According to the Social Care Institute for Excellence (SCIE 2013, p. 1):

Reablement is not effective unless care workers undergo specific training to understand the principles of delivering a reablement service.

Explicit acknowledgements of likely deterioration could be equally damaging, so that service users might not see the point of attempting the reablement goals. Again, careful management is required, with information being offered truthfully and in a timely way, without undue speculation as to outcomes. A goal-oriented approach requires flexibility to take account of fluctuations in health or social care contexts – for example, accidents such as falls, or deterioration in the service user's condition. On a practical level, goal-oriented approaches can be frustrated by delays in equipment arriving or delays in home modifications – for example, shower fitting or supply of a hoist to help get in and out of bed (Wilde and Glendinning 2012). Careful and timely communication and planning between health and social care professionals, as well as other agencies (for example, Age UK), should help to prevent this. Indeed, Glendinning and colleagues (2008, p. 55) suggest that an older person receiving services that deliver desired outcomes requires 'multiple, but nevertheless highly effective, channels of communication between users, service commissioners, contracts managers, care managers and both managers and front-line staff in provider organisations'.

Parsons and colleagues (2012) conducted a research study to determine the effect of using a goal facilitation tool with people on referral for home care reablement (New Zealand study on restorative home care). A randomised controlled trial with a total of 205 participants who showed significant improvements in health-related quality of life contended that:

There is broad agreement that HRQOL is the functional effect of a medical condition and/or its consequent therapy upon a patient. HRQOL is thus subjective and multidimensional, encompassing physical and occupational function, psychological state, social interaction and somatic sensation.

(ISOQOL 2015)

The researchers suggest that the significant improvements in HRQoL may have been because a higher proportion of individualised activities were tailored to a more successful identification of the person's goals (Parsons et al. 2012). This is an aspect that is highly relevant not only to individualised reablement planning but to the practical expertise of occupational therapists and their more advanced[2] **clinical reasoning skills** in the domain of occupation. The study places emphasis on other factors as well as physical activities of daily living. Aside from HRQoL these include autonomy, independence and social connectedness. A control group had a 'normal' home support package. There was no difference between groups in the percentage of services relating to domestic tasks, personal care or shopping. The main difference in services related to the proportion of individualised activities in the participants' support plans across the two groups. These were, for example, individualised walking or exercise programmes or other activities aimed at improving functional ability. In the intervention group, over 61% of the support plans described such individualised activities compared to 15% in the control group.

Parsons and colleagues (2012) suggest further research may be needed to investigate the impact of factors shown to affect the successful identification of goals. Individual client factors such as engagement and motivation, cultural considerations and ethnicity were key. The researchers also place emphasis on the assessors' and provider organisations' place in the process of reablement and goal setting. Crucially, one vital factor identified may include the experience and beliefs of the health or social care professionals working with the service user, as well as their professional background (Parsons et al. 2012).

The 'professional background' of the reablement worker

Wilde and Glendinning's (2012) study of users' and carers' views of reablement found that some service users felt a lack of professional expertise to help with specific aspects of reablement; one example cited was

---

[2] Not a particularly person-centred term but one that is understood by most professionals.

physiotherapists. This was in terms of mobility issues. It is interesting to speculate whether people trained as nurses or in a management role may be less proficient in reablement care and promoting independence than other health and social care professionals, such as OTs. Ryburn and colleagues (2009) found that reablement programmes vary widely in their structure, skill mix and the nature of the interventions. Typically, teams comprise OTs and social workers with some including 'physical therapists' (international term for physiotherapists). Nurses, however, are trained in health promotion, and evidence suggests that home visits to frail older adults involving health assessment, health education and empowerment strategies are associated with lowering ongoing health and community care costs (Markle-Reid et al. 2006). As part of its strategic plan, the Healthy Liverpool Programme has frailty units led by geriatricians and multidisciplinary teams in hospitals. These provide a link between hospital and community services with rapid discharge to the person's home. There is a clear link and thus a role for nurses here. This is especially so in the context of referrals to reablement services in the locality, part of the overall plan in the Liverpool project.

Box 4.2   The Healthy Liverpool Programme: Reablement service

'There will also be a redesigned community reablement service to create a modern integrated service that reduces the current over-reliance on hospital beds, providing care to more people in their own homes.'

'The Community Reablement Team will be commissioned to deliver a city-wide falls service within the community as a step up for general practice and an alternative to hospital for ambulance services.'

Source: **LCCG (2015, p. 42)**

A case example for this is with Sarah whose experience as a district nurse was challenged when she moved into a multidisciplinary rehabilitation team. Although not reablement, the same principles apply as activity within this domain is the vehicle for change. The positive side she found was that more time was allocated to each service user per visit (although the duration of visiting in the long term was shorter). This meant at a person level that facilitating and enabling the service user to increase their independence was valuable and constructive. But it did go against the grain of her previous experience in physically assisting 'patients' alongside relatively short visits. This contention however is illustrated in opposition in the comment below by a recreational therapist:

> I bring a different angle that they did not see, the more human side which they don't see because they're just so medical. The physio is doing the Get Up and Go, the OT is the Mini-Mental, the nurse is medication, and so on. I said, okay, but what does the patient want in all of this? ... So I bring that to the team and they know that it's true. But you've got to keep reminding them of that ...
>
> (Interview data: Hebblethwaite 2013, p. 26)

With the above points in mind all health and social care professionals need to be taught at undergraduate level the differences between working in reablement as opposed to care provision, but also intermediate care and rehabilitation services. This brings us to the role of support workers and formal and informal carers.

Support workers, formal and informal carers

The ways in which carers, both formal and informal, are trained and educated for reablement is critical if we are to avoid paternalistic 'doing for' or 'doing to' rather than 'doing with', encouraging and enabling autonomy. It is central in the effectiveness of achieving in reablement. Not only is good initial staff training essential, but also ongoing supervision, particularly for those for whom reablement is a change of role. Specifically, Rabiee and Glendinning (2011) indicate a need for improvement in work-based, multidisciplinary training, especially in counselling, group work and collaborative skills. Equally, staff need to be highly skilled in assessment and reassessment, constantly sensitive to small changes in the service user's condition or situation, if they are to maximise relevance and effectiveness. The importance of training in supporting workers is acknowledged as key, in that it requires a considerable paradigm shift from standard home care service delivery (Parsons et al. 2012). Some aspects require staff to learn 'to watch' and not 'interfere' when a service user is struggling to get something done (Rabiee and Glendinning 2011). One study suggests that staff with less experience in traditional home care work make better support workers in reablement services and are more likely to facilitate self-help (Rabiee and Glendinning 2011). There is, however, a paucity of further evidence to suggest that this is the case but this nonetheless suggests an important gap in current research. Ryburn (2009) reviews literature from Australia, the UK and the USA to provide an overview of the efficacy and effectiveness of **restorative approaches** towards home care for frail older adults. One conclusion is that a suitably skilled lead worker is required in order to avoid multiple assessment, promote co-ordination and preserve continuity of care. Support workers need to be better able to work in partnership with users and/or carers and to help people to come to terms with loss, disability, impairment and new ways of dealing with certain limitations. A more comprehensive discussion on the training and education of support workers follows in the next chapter.

The role of informal carers

Informal carers, such as partners, family and friends, need to be specifically aware of the purposes of reablement, and where possible should be encouraged to participate in the 'hands-off' process. This is particularly important when they live with the person needing care, as it is likely to be quicker and easier to 'do for' rather than watch a loved one struggle. Coupled with this is the previous family relationships, which are likely to be interdependent (one person has always relied on the other to do certain tasks and vice versa). This is very likely where the carer is the husband or wife, when lifelong habits may need to be altered. However, if informal carers are not taken into account in reablement programmes, this habitual behaviour can undermine the goal/s of service users working towards autonomy. Again, sensitive and timely communications may help to prevent this. Consider the following example which illustrates that the routine and habits of informal carers, prior to a reablement service, can undermine interventions. Wilde and Glendinning (2012) point out the potential for reablement services to help carers, by recognising the carers' own needs, but also by providing more advice on how informal carers can maximise and sustain a person's capabilities and move towards more autonomy.

Reflection Point 4.5 Influence of informal carers: Beth

Beth took pride in cooking and preparing meals for herself and her family but after her stroke, for a time, she was unable to cook in the way she preferred. Once Beth's mobility improved, she was keen to get back to cooking from scratch, as she felt it was healthier and tastier. Nonetheless, informal carers insisted on bringing her microwave ready meals which she disliked. Her two daughters argued that it was easier for Beth to manage these, and that if she had to cook from basic ingredients she would not eat properly. Beth felt that this decision had been taken from her, and being unable to do her own shopping was unable to do anything about it.

Student Activity 4.2   Supporting informal carers

Think about the following response from Beth's daughter, Ruth, following a reablement support group and workshop for informal carers.

'Since her stroke, mum's needs and wishes vary on a daily basis, depending on whether she's having a good day or a not so good a day. Things like choosing what she's going to wear, helping her fasten her bra, and making choices about what she's going to have for breakfast are very much easier to do myself. I sometimes have to pick up her clothes if they fall and I used to take them out of the cupboard. But mum has always been an independent person and although it takes longer... giving her the chance to do things for herself is helping her regain that independence. I know she feels better about herself. I always try to encourage her, but it's hard at times ... I mean watching her struggle ... I often feel very guilty just standing there and I have to zip it (laughs) ... that's hard.'

Q. Do you think providing specific support groups and workshops for informal carers might be useful? Write down your answer:

_____

_____

_____

_____

Q. In your response, did you clarify why you thought it was/was not useful? If you didn't go back and be more specific.

Q. When re-examining Ruth's statement earlier would you agree with the following?

1. Ruth has a better understanding now of how to enable proactive facilitation.

2. Ruth's new approach to reablement is more supportive.

3. Beth is regaining autonomy with Ruth's more discreet assistance.

Q. Are you confident that the family will be better able to support Beth when the reablement intervention ends?

The role of direct payments in promoting autonomy

Although reablement itself does not fall into the category of being costed for the first six weeks – that is, the service user having to be means-tested to assess if payment is required – continuing care following a reablement period may well do. Arguably one way of preserving and encouraging autonomy is to offer the service user 'direct payments' (DP), so that they can choose their care depending on their needs. This may also be outsourced to a provider with experience of 'enabling' or at least with a good grounding in the reablement ethos. Through DP people purchase their own care rather than having to depend on social care assessors/workers in local authorities. In brief, advocates of direct payments indicate that DPs facilitate people to live in the ways that *they* choose to live, rather than being given services to match preconceived assumptions about what is needed and how individuals should live. DPs provide greater flexibility and reliability over when, how and who provides the support that people need (Halliwell and Glendinning 1998 cited in Spandler 2004). For instance, people want to get up in the morning at a time of their choosing, not when service providers can make it. This can sometimes mean an early morning call at 7.30am or at the other extreme 10.30am! However, DPs are not without issues, with limitations in terms of bureaucracy and administration, which may lead to them being inappropriate for frail, elderly people. Their place in reablement therefore needs to be considered carefully when weighing up the prospect for self-determination and independence for service users. This is again illustrated in the following comment: *'Well now I've been told I've got this budget but it's got to start next week! They want me to spend it on this new agency of carers. I'm sure they're very good, but I want to do other things with it too'* (Pitts et al. 2011, p. 7).

Another offshoot of this, from a person-centred perspective is that personal budgets provide opportunity for social interaction or reablement. This was discussed in Chapter 2. Social contexts are often missing in goal setting with primary needs such as PADL and DADL given more priority. Discussing outcomes-focused social care services, Glendinning and colleagues (2008) found that while intermediate and reablement developed outcome-focused services, later maintenance care was more fragmented, as the capacity of home care services to address maintenance outcomes was limited. Outcomes proposed in a Green Paper (DH 2005) placed an emphasis on choice and control, as well as improved quality of life. The increased use of DP is therefore advocated; however, in 2006 its use unfortunately for older people remained low. In fact, more recently Ryan (2016) reports that due to drastic cuts in social care funding individuals have been left without support, often older parents of adults living with them at home. In addition, the report from the Independent Living Survey (In Control, 2016, n.p.) adds that concerning choice and control:

Just under half (48%) of all respondents reported that the choice and control they enjoyed over their support was poor or very poor.

And concerning quality of life and well-being:

> Well over half (58%) of respondents reported that their quality of life had reduced or reduced significantly over the past 12 months.

Home Instead, in the north-west's private sector, provides home care for help with domestic and personal care. Of more interest here, however, is its emphasis on companionship and the recognition of people's social needs. The organisation's care staff develop relationships with many older people whose families are not in proximity. They do this with thought. For example, in one instance help was sought to enable a woman in her 80s to keep her dog – a very much loved companion. This was achieved by seeking external agency support. In 2015 the partnership working on a project between Home Instead, Wirral University Teaching Hospital NHS Foundation Trust and the University of Chester was recognised in a nomination for the HRH Prince of Wales Integrated Care Award (2015). Although not the overall winners, this positive experience led to further work in getting nursing students to experience longer term placements with Home Instead and to appreciate what a good model of care might look like. Importantly, students are encouraged to take up spoke placements (drop-out days from the main placement site) while hospital ward-based. This enables them to see the continuum of care but with a difference – one that addresses some very pertinent social or emotive needs: a relationship-led care model. Home Instead is an organisation that is ideally placed to facilitate reablement because there is already an existing 'do with' as well as 'do for' ethos from support staff. Outsourcing was discussed in Chapter 3 and this is an area which may grow and develop as evidence of effectiveness accumulates. Essentially, organisations like Home Instead place good-quality training as a priority in their overall workforce development. This is consistently identified as key in reablement service development and the current available literature:

> We have the potential to help alter the common perception that all social care is of poor quality. And from a health economics perspective, we hope it will pave the way for more cost effective care in the community, with more timely and effective discharge of elderly patients from hospital.
>
> (Chester Chronicle 2015)

Intensity and duration of reablement services

There is some discussion about what the 'optimum' duration of reablement services should be. How is the transition from the intense reablement programme to no support or diminished support managed? Some service users and carers express concern over the 'handover' when reablement finishes (Trappes-Lomax and Hawton 2012). Reverting to traditional agency services could undo some or all of the autonomy gained if these services do not understand the conceptual basis and ethos of reablement. Trappes-Lomax and Hawton (2012) go on to suggest that care pathways should be extended beyond discharge, involving service users and carers more closely in discharge planning. Co-production was discussed in Chapter 2. The commissioning process should support self-care and sustain informal care networks, which should improve quality of life and may also help to reduce unnecessary admissions to hospital or long-term care (Trappes-Lomax and Hawton 2012). We should not be hearing from service users that they are confused by the aim of reablement. Nor that they have been left distraught because they think that formal care will be completely removed – forever! An example of this can be seen in the following statement taken from Pitts and colleagues (2011):

> *I've been told these carers are finishing soon, but they don't know yet what will happen after that. I hope they don't send a bunch of new folk. I'm sick of all these strangers in my house.*

This chapter has explored features of dependency and independence, or otherwise oft-cited 'autonomy', in the reablement process. Although more research is needed, it is clear that there are certain aspects of managing care and reablement that make the process more effective in facilitating autonomy. In particular, the need for good planning, goal setting, communication and training have been identified, and the roles of both formal and informal carers in facilitating independence and avoiding dependency have been discussed. Equally, the definitions and perceptions of dependence and autonomy are crucial in supporting care that is aware and considerate for both service users and carers themselves. At the same time, it is critical to step back and actively listen. While keeping an open mind and a keenness to facilitate the service user in identifying what types of activities they associate with autonomy, it is essential to establish the meaningfulness of desired goals. All these conditions should be apparent. There is now a need to move from the idea that we are 'experts' by default – whether professionals or seasoned support workers – to one of co-productive partnership with those we serve.

Summary

➢ Reablement requires moving away from ideas of 'incompetence' or 'lack of ability' to individualised self-determination.

➢ The ethos of reablement requires a 'hands-off' culture 'to do and be – with support'.

➢ A lack of autonomy can lead to situations of learned helplessness, which is often perpetuated by the way services create dependent relationships.

➢ How we communicate with a person, their families and partners, and equally, with each other, needs more thought. It is crucial to the success of reablement.

➢ The involvement of families is as important as the individual in our care, whether we are professionals or support workers. This is especially the case when informal carers are involved in 'doing for' their relative or have been in the past.

➢ Specific reablement training, which is a repeated theme throughout many chapters, needs to be carefully considered, with more investment including time.

Recommended listening, reading and additional learning

BBC4. (2015) The secret lives of carers. New Models of Care. [Online Player Radio] Available at: http://www.bbc.co.uk/programmes/b06qjqcv (Accessed 2 January 2016).

HAMMEL, K. W. (2006) *Perspectives on disability and rehabilitation: Contesting assumptions; challenging practice.* Edinburgh: Churchill Livingstone.

SCIE (SOCIAL CARE INSTITUTE OF EXCELLENCE). (2016) *What is personalisation and where did it come from.* E-learning resource. Available at: http://www.scie.org.uk/publications/elearning/personalisation/index.asp (Accessed 2 February 2014).

THOMPSON, N. (2012) *Anti-discriminatory practice: equality, diversity and social justice.* Basingstoke: Palgrave Macmillan.

References

AGE UK. (2014) Loneliness in later life. Evidence review. Available at: https://www.ageuk.org.uk/globalassets/age-uk/documents/reports-and-publications/reports-and-briefings/health--wellbeing/rb_june15_lonelines_in_later_life_evidence_review.pdf (Accessed 12 December 2017).

BARNES, C. (2014) Disability, disability studies, and the academy. In J. Swain, S. French, C. Barnes & C. Thomas (eds) *Disabling barriers – Enabling environments*. London: Sage, pp. 17–23.

BARNES, C., MERCER, G. & SHAKESPEARE, T. (1999) Exploring disability: A sociological introduction. Cambridge: Polity Press.

BARTON, L. & OLIVER, M. (1997) *Disability studies: Past, present and future*. Leeds: The Disability Press.

CAMERON, C. (2014) Developing an affirmative model of disability and impairment. In J. Swain, S. French, C. Barnes & C. Thomas (eds) *Disabling barriers – Enabling environments*. London: Sage, pp. 24–29.

CHESTER CHRONICLE. (2015) *University of Chester lecturers nominated for Nursing Times award. Communication*. Available at: http://www.chesterchronicle. co.uk/news/university-chester-lecturers-nominated-nursing-9886347 (Accessed 3 October 2015).

COMMISSION FOR HEALTHCARE AUDIT AND INSPECTION. (2006) *Living well in later life: Review of progress against the National Service Framework for Older People*. Available at: http://www.scie.org.uk/publications/guides/guide15/ files/livingwellinlaterlife-fullreport.pdf?res=true (Accessed 24 February 2014).

CORDEN, A. & HIRST, M. (2011) Partner care at the end-of-life: Identity, language and characteristics. *Ageing and Society*, vol. 31, no. 2, 217–242.

DARZI, A. (2008) *High Quality Care for All: NHS Next Stage Review*, Final Report. London: Department of Health.

DH (DEPARTMENT OF HEALTH). (2001) *The National Service Framework for Older People*. Available at: https://www.gov.uk/government/uploads/system/ uploads/attachment_data/file/198033/National_Service_Framework_for_ Older_People.pdf (Accessed 2 June 2013).

DH (DEPARTMENT OF HEALTH). (2005) *Independence, well-being and choice: Our vision for the future of social care for adults in England*. Available at: https:// www.gov.uk/government/uploads/system/uploads/attachment_data/ file/272101/6499.pdf (Accessed 2 May 2014).

DH (DEPARTMENT OF HEALTH). (2007) *Putting people first: a shared vision and commitment to the transformation of adult social care*. Available at: http:// webarchive.nationalarchives.gov.uk/20130107105354/http:/www.dh.gov.uk/ en/Publicationsandstatistics/Publications/PublicationsPolicyAndGuidance/ DH_081118 (Accessed 2 February 2013).

FINE, M. & GLENDINNING, C. (2005) Dependence, independence or interdependence? Revisiting the concepts of 'care' and 'dependency'. *Ageing and Society*, vol. 25, 601–621.

FRANCIS, J., FISHER, M. & RUTTER, D. (2011) *Reablement: a cost-effective route to better outcomes*. Research Briefing, London: SCIE.

GLENDINNING, C., CLARKE, S., HARE, P., MADDISON, J. & NEWBRONNER, L. (2008) Progress and problems in developing outcomes-focussed social care services for older people in England. *Health and Social Care in the Community*, vol. 16, no. 1, 54–63.

GOBLE, C. (2014) Dependence, independence and normality. In J. Swain, S. French, C. Barnes & C. Thomas (eds) *Disabling barriers – Enabling environments*. London: Sage, pp. 31–36.

HEBBLETHWAITE, S. (2013) "I think that it could work but..." Tensions between the theory and practice of person-centred and relationship-centred care. *Therapeutic Recreation Journal*, vol. 47, no. 1, 13–34.

IN CONTROL. (2014) *About us.* Registered Charity. Available at: http://www.in-control.org.uk/about-us.aspx (Accessed 8 June 2014).

IN CONTROL. (2016) *Report on the Independent Living Survey 2016.* Available at: http://www.in-control.org.uk/news/in-control-news/report-on-the-independent-living-survey-2016.aspx (Accessed 12 December 2017).

ISOQOL (INTERNATIONAL SOCIETY FOR QUALITY OF LIFE RESEARCH). (2015) *What is health-related quality of life research?* Available at: http://www.Isoqol.org/about-isoqol/what-is-health-related-quality-of-life-research (Accessed 12 January 2015).

KENDRICK, M. (2000) *Some observations on what on person can do in human services. Sharing the Road in 1999.* Proceedings of the 1999 Conference for Direct Support Workers Education. Brisbane: Montgomery C.B ASSID (QLD).

LCCG (LIVERPOOL CLINICAL COMMISSIONING GROUP). (2015) *The healthy Liverpool programme.* Available at: http://www.healthyliverpool.nhs.uk/ (Accessed 10 July 2015).

LEWIN, G., DE SAN MIGUEL, K., KNUIMAN, M., ALAN, J., BOLDY, D., HENDRIE D. & VANDERMEULEN, S. (2013) A randomised controlled trial of the Home Independence Program, an Australian restorative home-care programme for older adults. *Health and Social Care in the Community*, vol. 21, no. 1, 69–78.

MARKLE-REID, M., WEIR, R., BROWNE, G., ROBERTS, J., GAFNI, A. & HENDERSON, S. (2006) Health Promotion for frail older home care clients. *Journal of Advanced Nursing*, vol. 54, no. 3, 381–395.

MARKS, D. (1999) Disability: Controversial debates and psychosocial perspectives. London: Routledge.

MUNRO, K. & ELDER-WOODWARD, J. (1992) *Independent living.* Edinburgh: Churchill Livingston.

NOLAN, M. R., DAVIES, S., BROWN, J., KEADY, J. & NOLAN, J. (2004) Beyond 'person-centred' care: a new vision for gerontological nursing. *International Journal of Older People Nursing in association with Journal of Clinical Nursing*, vol. 13, no. 3a, 45–53.

PANORAMA. (2015) NHS: *The perfect storm.* Available at: http://www.bbc.co.uk/programmes/b05y3fcb (Aired 3 June 2015 on BBC1 iPlayer).

PARSONS, J., ROUSE, P., ROBINSON, E. M., SHERIDAN, N. & CONNOLLY, M. J. (2012) Goal setting as a feature of homecare services for older people: does it make a difference? *Age and ageing*, vol. 41, 24–29.

PITTS, J., SANDERSON, H., WEBSTER, A. & SKELHORN, L. (2011) *A new reablement journey.* Ambrey Associates and Helen Sanderson Associates. Available at: https://www.centreforwelfarereform.org/uploads/attachment/267/a-new-reablement-journey.pdf (Accessed 12 December 2017).

RABIEE, P. & GLENDINNING, C. (2011) Organisation and delivery of home care re-ablement: What makes a difference? *Health and Social Care in the Community*, vol. 19, no. 5, 495–503.

RYAN, F. (2016) The right to choose your own care is the latest casualty of council cuts. *The Guardian*, 7 December. Available at: https://www.theguardian.com/society/2016/dec/07/personal-budget-disabled-funding-cuts-social-care (Accessed 12 December 2017).

RYBURN, B., WELLS, Y. & FOREMAN, P. (2009) Enabling independence: Restorative approaches to home care provision for frail older adults. *Health and Social Care in the Community*, vol. 17, no. 3, 225–234.

SARAGA, T. (1998) *Embodying the social: Constructions of difference*. London: Routledge.

SCHMITT, J., AKROYD, K. & BURKE, L. (2012) Perceptions of physiotherapy students of a person-centred approach in rehabilitation. *International Journal of Therapy and Rehabilitation*, vol. 19, no. 1, 23–30.

SCIE (SOCIAL CARE INSTITUTE FOR EXCELLENCE). (2013) SCIE Guide 49 'Maximising the potential of reablement', London: SCIE.

SPANDLER, H. (2004) Friend or Foe? Towards a critical assessment of direct payments. *Critical Social Policy*, vol. 24, 187–209.

SUMSION, T. & SMYTH, G. (2000) Barriers to client-centredness and their resolution. *Canadian Journal of Occupational Therapy*, vol. 67, no. 1, 15–21.

THOMPSON, N. (1998) Promoting equality: Challenging discrimination and oppression in the human services. New York: Palgrave.

THOMPSON, N. (2011) *Promoting equality: Working with diversity and difference*. Basingstoke: Palgrave Macmillan.

THOMPSON, N. (2012) *Partnership and empowerment*. SOCIAL WORK/ SOCIAL CARE AND MEDIA. Available at: https://swscmedia.wordpress.com/2012/12/10/partnership-and-empowerment-by-dr-neil-thompson/ (Accessed 12 December 2017).

TRAPPES-LOMAX, T. & HAWTON, A. (2012) The user voice: Older people's experiences of reablement and rehabilitation. *Journal of Integrated Care*, vol. 20, no. 3, 181–194.

TURNER, A. (1997) *Occupational therapy and physical dysfunction: Principles, skills and practice*. Edinburgh: Churchill Livingston.

UPIAS (UNION OF THE PHYSICALLY IMPAIRED AGAINST SEGREGATION) and THE DISABILITY ALLIANCE. (1975) *Fundamental Principles of Disability*. Available at: http://www.disability.co.uk/fundamental-principles-disability (Accessed 24 November 2017).

WILDE, A. & GLENDINNING, C. (2012) If they're helping me, then how can I be independent? The perceptions and experience of users of home-care re-ablement services. *Health and Social Care in the Community*, vol. 20, no. 6, 583–590.

WILLIAMS, S. J. (2005) Parsons revisited: From the sick role to ...? Health – *An Interdisciplinary Journal for the Social Study of Health, Illness and Medicine*, vol. 9, no. 2, 123–144.

5

Reablement and Support Workers

L. Dibsdall, A. Clampin and H. M. Chapman

Chapter outline

Support workers are key to the delivery of reablement services as they are the people who work on a day-to-day basis with service users. Support workers may join reablement teams without any experience in working in health and social care. More commonly, support workers move into reablement teams from therapy assistant roles or from working in a home care service. These support workers bring a wealth of experience to the role, but differences in both the process and the outcome of reablement and home care can offset the benefits of this experience. Reablement is a change in approach to care from being 'task-led' to a 'doing with', **person-centred** and **outcomes-based** approach. This holistic view of working with people who use these services has been largely welcomed by support workers who enjoy supporting them to do more for themselves.

This chapter will consider some key skills and techniques used by support workers in reablement services, such as use of equipment, activity analysis and energy conservation. Support workers need appropriate training and education in reablement so that practice is meaningful, and the concept of reablement is clearly understood and articulated. This is fundamental to an inclusive approach to interacting with the service user, enabling them to grow in confidence and autonomy, and engage in the process of reablement. Suggested topics for inclusion in reablement training are included in this chapter and it is argued that occupational therapists (OT) are suitably experienced, and well placed, to provide this training. Before reading any further, you may want to recap on the concept discussed in Chapter 1 in the section 'Defining occupation, activity and task (OAT) for reablement interventions'.

Chapter objectives

By the end of this chapter you should be able to:

➤ Outline the development of the reablement support worker role

➤ Compare and contrast 'doing to' and 'doing with' support worker approaches

➤ Explain the role of the support worker

➤ Evaluate equipment and reablement techniques support workers may use

➤ Describe the training requirements for being a support worker

➤ Consider the opportunities and challenges of being a support worker

The development of the support worker role in reablement

Government guidance in England has focused on the personalisation of services and the development of preventative and reablement services within health and social care over a number of years (DH 2007, 2009, 2010) and most recently in the Care Act 2014 (DH 2014). The importance of person-centred working and prevention services are mirrored in the legislation for Wales, the Social Services and Well-being (Wales) Act 2014 (Welsh Assembly Government 2014), in April 2016, and are also inherent in existing legislation for Northern Ireland and Scotland (Northern Ireland Assembly 2009; Scottish Parliament 2013).

Personalisation in health and social care involves giving people more choice and control. It focuses on service users' goals, strengths and preferences (SCIE 2010). Reablement supports personalisation as a service working with people to support them to achieve their health and well-being outcomes. While there have been calls for a common framework on reablement (Bridges and James 2012), reablement services are structured and funded differently in different areas of the UK and around the world. Many local authorities in the UK refocused their existing in-house home care services into reablement services (Allen and Glasby 2010). Some services have developed as new integrated health and social care services or they may be commissioned as being service-led either by health or social care. Support workers occupy a pivotal role in reablement services since they spend the most time working with people in their own homes. Support workers often join teams from different backgrounds bringing valuable experience to the role.

From therapy assistant to reablement support worker

Support workers may have previously worked in health or social care as OT, physiotherapy (PT) or rehabilitation assistants. Therapy or rehabilitation assistants typically work with people in a hospital setting, an outpatient setting or within services users' own homes. The therapy assistant's role is to implement therapy support plans agreed between with the service user and an OT or PT. The therapy support plan would involve working with the person to participate in daily living activities including mobility. This includes supporting him or her in practising skills, and the use of equipment to facilitate more autonomy. This experience in enabling people to undertake daily activities, following a therapy support plan, is mirrored in the focus of reablement in supporting people to meet their own outcomes, rather than carrying out tasks for them. It is not clear how many therapy assistants have moved into reablement services as support workers.

Student Activity 5.1   Working with people in hospitals versus their own home setting

Identify the key differences between working with people in a hospital setting and working with people in their own homes.

Hospital Setting	Own Home

Therapy assistants will have had experience in being supervised by therapy staff and regularly communicating information to the therapist on the progress of the service user towards their goals (Barnes and Frock 2003). This skill is essential to working in an enabling way and regularly reviewing the effectiveness of the reablement intervention in terms of service user outcomes.

From home care worker to reablement support worker

The role of home care services in the UK has changed considerably since its beginnings as 'home help' for older people after the Second World War. 'Home help' was provided by the local authority social services department and largely involved providing domestic support in the home, such as with cleaning and shopping. The closure of hospital wards for older people and the focus on supporting people in their own homes saw the change from 'home help' services to 'home care' services (Sinclair, Gibbs and Hicks 2000). Home care services include support with personal care, for example with using the toilet and having a wash.

As home carers visit a number of people in the community, a timed care plan is agreed between the service user and the home care service. This care plan has been described as a 'task-led' care plan where support workers complete tasks for people within the specified time. These types of care plans have also been described as a 'doing to' approach to care. Some support workers have felt obliged to do things for service users as it is quicker and easier within the time given (Baker et al. 2001).

Support workers who have previously been home carers bring experience of working independently with people in their own homes to the reablement team. Support workers have been central to the development of reablement services in some areas. In Leicestershire, workers in the home care service asserted that if they only had 30 minutes to visit someone at home, then they were limited to having to do things for service users. It was recognised by managers that doing tasks for service users led to loss of their self-care skills and dependency on services. The initial comments from the home care workers led to the reconfiguration of the existing home care service into HART, Leicester's Home Assessment and Reablement Team (Norris 2008). Staff, rather than providing care, work with service users to complete daily living activities (ADL) and the focus is on meeting service users' outcomes rather than completing care tasks.

Reablement: A change in approach to care for support workers

Reablement is typically short-term, focused support. It is a move from a task-led 'doing to' approach to a 'doing with' approach. The reablement support plan is based on service users' outcomes. It involves working in a person-centred way, where the focus of care is based on the needs of the person, as discussed and negotiated with the reablement team. This contrasts with the traditional task-centred care of completing washing and dressing, feeding or other checklist outcomes. Instead of working on

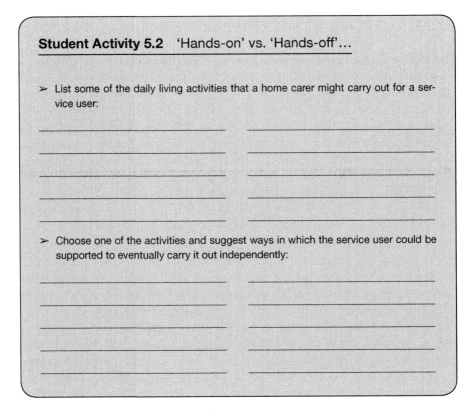

Student Activity 5.2   'Hands-on' vs. 'Hands-off'...

➤ List some of the daily living activities that a home carer might carry out for a service user:

➤ Choose one of the activities and suggest ways in which the service user could be supported to eventually carry it out independently:

a care plan stating 'prepare breakfast for Mr Jones', a reablement support plan may include an outcome of 'Mr Jones will prepare his breakfast'. Information on how to work with Mr Jones to enable him to prepare his breakfast will be shared in the reablement support plan. Support workers may be given an approximate length of time for visiting a service user. In many settings support workers can be flexible with the length of time they spend with service users. For example, they may stay longer with one service user to enable them to do as much as they can for themselves at their own pace. Support workers then only need to report to their supervisor if they are likely to be with a service user for more than a set period of time (McLeod and Mair 2009; Rabiee and Glendinning 2011).

Agreeing outcomes with service users is essential to successful reablement as it places the service user in control (for more on control, see Chapter 7). Working in a reabling way has been described as requiring a change in mindset for the whole team (Care Services Efficiency Delivery 2007). The Office for Public Management, an organisation of independent facilitators, has completed successful workshops with commissioners and staff on 'behaviour change and reablement', looking at how to ensure behaviour change is sustained following a period of reablement (Bunnin 2011).

Some support workers find the change in approach of reablement services challenging. Research has shown that some support workers who have transferred into reablement services from home care services have found standing back difficult. Support workers were concerned about seeing a service user have difficulty undertaking an activity on their own. In other settings managers have found that new workers to reablement services accepted a more encouraging approach more readily (Rabiee et al. 2009).

> *'I love being more involved with service users, looking at what people can do'*
> *(Reablement support worker)*

The change of approach in reablement services has clearly been welcomed by some staff. Support workers have commented that they 'relished the challenge' to work in a different way (McLeod and Mair 2009). Working in reablement services has led to increased job satisfaction for support workers (Office for Public Management 2010). A comparison study of support workers from home care services and support workers in reablement services was undertaken as part of a larger study of reablement, or **restorative care** as it is known in New Zealand. The study reported a reduced turnover of staff in the restorative care service. In the restorative care service 17.9% (5 out of 28) people left the service. In the home care service 42.5% (17 out of 40) people left their job over a 14-month period (King et al. 2012). The increased job satisfaction of support workers in the restorative care service was attributed to increased support from co-ordinators, and training and flexibility in the activities they undertook with service users, such as accompanying a service user to do activities outside their home.

Team managers have praised the 'can do' attitude of their reablement support workers in motivating service users to do more for themselves (Care Services Efficiency Delivery 2007). The attitude of support workers is essential to providing high-quality support. Ebenstein (1998) interviewed six support workers who were identified by social workers as being outstanding at work. The support workers identified patience, compassion and respect as key elements of working with older people. At this point you may want to refer back to Chapter 2 and the section on 'The appropriate culture of compassion'.

The carers discussed using music and puzzle activities to engage with older people. When discussing job satisfaction, the support workers highlighted working closely with service users and seeing an improvement in service users' lives as key features to their job satisfaction. Reablement is a service that aims to improve the lives of service users and is an exciting opportunity for support workers.

A change in approach for service users

Reablement is a change in approach from being a professional-led service to being more person-centred and so communication between support workers and service users is essential. Support workers are the members of the team who spend most time with service users and usually start to build rapport from the initial assessment onwards. Listening to older people is important as service users often have ideas on what they could do to continue their participation in daily living activities. A study of older people in New Zealand identified a number of strategies older people used to help them continue to complete ordinary activities. They described fixing bags to a walking aid, using a taxi to come home from the shops, keeping pans on the hob and eating ready meals as strategies for making meal preparation easier (Hocking, Murphy and Reed 2011).

It has been recognised that service users who have had support from home care services in the past can have an expectation that support workers will 'do for' them (Rabiee et al. 2009). Reablement is typically a short-term service and service users may be concerned about not having support in the long term. To manage expectations, it is important for support workers to be clear with service users on their role as a reablement support worker. Sometimes there may still be a need for formal care support when some areas of difficulty continue. Support workers can use their skills in encouragement and motivation to demonstrate to service users that they are able to do more for themselves. Not all service users have the same attitude. Lena Borell, in her keynote address to the European Congress of Occupational Therapy, relayed that during interviews a group of older women in Sweden wished for a 'doing with' assistant. The role of the 'doing with' assistant was to help the older women with daily living activities supporting older people to remain engaged in daily living occupations as much as possible (Borell 2008). The 'doing with' assistant is consistent with the ethos of reablement services and demonstrates that older people do wish to be supported to undertake their daily living activities as opposed to having someone do their activities for them. You may want to refer to Chapter 2 at this point for a recap on where the ideas of 'doing with' come from and the associated paradigm; see the section on 'Personalisation'.

Being a reablement support worker

Reablement support workers enable service users to be independent at the level of autonomy that is deemed right for the individual referred to the service. Reablement support workers need to utilise skills in observation and 'standing back' to understand service users' potential (Rabiee and Glendinning 2011).

Student Activity 5.3   Individual meaning of independence

Q. What does independence mean to you?

_____

_____

_____

Q. What activities do you prefer to carry out unaided?

_____

_____

_____

Q. How would you feel if you lost your independence in those activities?

_____

_____

_____

Independence means different things to different people. It may mean being independent on one particular task, such as brushing teeth. It may mean having choice and control over what tasks other people support a service user with, so the service user has the energy to complete other tasks that they wish to do independently. This type of autonomy was discussed in the previous chapter.

Reablement support workers may use a variety of techniques while working with service users, including breaking down an activity (**activity analysis**), **backward chaining** (carrying out the activity starting with the last part, to gain immediate reward for effort), **energy conservation** (ensuring that the service user has sufficient energy to carry out the tasks that they most want independence in) and use of equipment to make activities achievable. Training for support workers in these areas is essential to ensure support workers have the knowledge and skills to work effectively with service users. Again, the fundamentals of activity were discussed in Chapter 1 alongside another example of energy conservation.

Equipment

Service users may be provided with equipment and adaptations to support them to complete daily living activities, as part of the reablement service. For example, a service user may be given a perching stool in the kitchen to enable him or her to sit at a worktop to prepare food, if they do not have a table and chair in the kitchen. In some services, support workers are trained to assess for basic pieces of equipment. Table 5.1 is a non-exhaustive list of a number of items of equipment and their features.

Equipment for complex needs has to be assessed by an OT (Newbronner et al. 2007). With specific training support workers can become trusted assessors (DLF 2015) with the autonomy to prescribe equipment and the skills of adequate reporting and sharing of information with interdisciplinary team members. Whether a support worker is trained to assess for basic equipment or not, they need to have a good awareness of the types of equipment that can be provided. This will

Table 5.1   Examples of basic equipment used in reablement services

Equipment	Features of equipment
Shower seat – can be freestanding or fixed to the wall	*Standing to shower can be tiring; sitting on a seat can reduce fatigue for a service user.*
Raised toilet seat	*It is more difficult to get up from a low seat. For taller people a raised toilet seat can support them to stand more easily.*
Kettle tipper – existing kettle sits inside the tipper	*Full kettles are heavy; kettles in tippers can be filled with water from a jug. Using the tipper to pour the kettle can be safer for those with a tremor or limited hand or arm strength.*
Vegetable basket – a wire basket placed in a saucepan	*Saucepans filled with hot water are heavy and put people at risk of scalding if spilt when carrying. Cooking vegetables in a basket in the saucepan enables the service user to lift out only the vegetables. Vegetables in the basket are lighter than the water in the saucepan and therefore easier to lift.*
Long-handled shoe horn	*The long handle supports people who find it difficult to reach down to put on their shoes.*

enable support workers to confidently demonstrate how the equipment is used with service users and, in some cases, prescribe it. Training also helps support workers to identify when a referral to another member of the team is necessary. This might be to complete an assessment of need additional to those that are being met that could benefit the service user.

Techniques used in reablement

Activity analysis

The member of the team who develops the reablement support plan with the service user, typically an OT, may complete an activity analysis on the task that the service user wants to achieve independently. Activity analysis involves considering the task in relation to the service user: identifying physical, cognitive, sensory, social and emotional skills needed to complete the task and also the importance of cultural differences relating to the task (Kielhofner and Forsyth 2009). This activity analysis, carried out by the OT with the service user, forms the basis for the support worker's intervention with the service user.

Activity analysis is helpful in achieving service user-led outcomes. For example, Mr Jones, who has Parkinson's disease, states that his memory is not as good as it used to be. He has difficulties mobilising and experiences tremor carrying out everyday activities. Mr Jones would like to be able to make a sandwich for his lunch autonomously. The OT analyses the task of making a sandwich in relation to Mr Jones' need. Mr Jones enjoys jam sandwiches. Table 5.2 illustrates the tasks associated with making a jam sandwich. Considering the activity analysis outlined, the support worker may initially walk with Mr Jones to the kitchen and prompt him to get all the items he needs to prepare his sandwich. Some items (butter) may be too low in the fridge so he might be asked to keep these on higher shelves. In some cases, funding can be provided to make a plinth to raise the fridge to a better height.

The support worker might encourage Mr Jones to consider sitting at his table to prepare his sandwich to reduce the effort of standing to complete the task (energy conservation). Mr Jones may need verbal prompting for several sessions to sit at the table as this would be a new routine for him. The support worker would verbally prompt Mr Jones at each stage of the process of making the sandwich if required. If he had trouble spreading butter and jam a small flat device with prongs might be used to stabilise the bread. The support worker would ask Mr Jones if he wanted to eat alone or if he would like the support worker to sit with him. This reflects the person-centred approach following Mr Jones' preferences, as his activity analysis indicated that he liked to eat alone; he is nonetheless given the choice.

Table 5.2 Activity analysis: Making a jam sandwich

Skill	Analysis
Physical	Mr Jones will need to walk to the kitchen to gather items to make his sandwich. Mr Jones may have difficulty standing for the length of time needed to make a sandwich.
	Twisting off a jar lid involves using both hands and Mr Jones may have difficulty gripping the jar due to his tremor. Mr Jones has difficulty holding one piece of bread still while gripping a knife with the other hand to spread his jam.
Cognitive	Making a sandwich involves following a number of steps in a certain order. Mr Jones may not remember where he keeps his jam.
Sensory	Mr Jones has no sensory problems. He can feel the knife in his hand and the pressure required to spread the jam on the bread.
Social	Mr Jones usually prefers to eat alone.
Emotional	Making a sandwich may test Mr Jones' patience if it takes him several times to get the jam out of the jar due to his tremor. He may initially have feelings of helplessness if he is unable to carry out the task. He may have a greater sense of achievement when he is able to make his own sandwich.

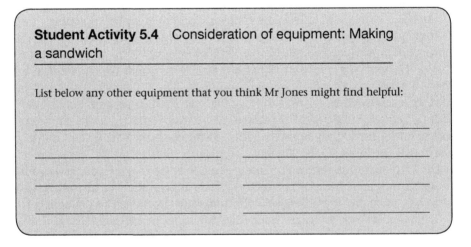

Student Activity 5.4   Consideration of equipment: Making a sandwich

List below any other equipment that you think Mr Jones might find helpful:

_____   _____

_____   _____

_____   _____

_____   _____

Backward chaining

A support worker may be asked to use a backward chaining method to motivate and enable service users to complete a particular activity. In backward chaining the task is analysed and broken down into a series of steps. The support worker completes most of the steps of the task and the service user completes the last step (Schreibman 1985). For example, if a person is being supported to dress independently, the support worker may help them to choose a jumper and put it over the service user's head, then support them to put one arm into the sleeve. The service user is then prompted to put their other arm into the remaining sleeve. With this method the service user gets a sense of achievement from having finished a task, increasing their motivation to persist with the activity. The service user is encouraged to complete more of the preceding steps of the activity until they can complete the whole activity independently.

Energy conservation

Many older people experience fatigue (Yu, Lee and Man 2010). This can be pain-related as well as associated with stiff joints, limited movement for one reason or another or high levels of **spasticity** or **clonus**. Fatigue can be a major factor impeding the ability to carry out activities that people need and want to do. As part of a reablement programme, support workers may be asked to encourage services users to think about energy conservation. This is a term which is used to describe different strategies that can be used to manage fatigue (Dreiling 2009). If support workers have an awareness of helpful strategies, they can subsequently facilitate people to make small changes so that they have the energy to complete meaningful activities. Dreiling (2009) suggests **six strategies** to enable this.

The **first strategy** is keeping a journal. This involves service users considering how much energy individual activities take on a daily basis to gain an understanding of how different activities affect people.

The **next two strategies** are to prioritise and plan. Once service users have used a journal to understand their fatigue, they can prioritise the activities that are important to them and plan their week accordingly. For example, if it is important for the service user to be able to go out to eat with their family, and they know that activity will be tiring, they may plan not to complete any other activities at home before or after the meal.

The **fourth strategy** is pacing. This involves achieving a balance between activity and rest. Support workers working with people with fatigue should encourage them to rest regularly before they become fatigued. Regular short breaks can reduce fatigue.

The **fifth strategy** is posture. A service user may have had an assessment by a physiotherapist if they experience poor posture. Support workers can encourage service users to think about posture in relation to their fatigue. For example, using a long-handled shoe horn requires less effort than reaching down to put shoes on. Pushing a wheeled trolley (or asking a shop assistant to assist with this) in the supermarket rather than carrying a basket uses less muscle strength, conserving energy.

The final strategy concerns the environment. Support workers can work with service users to reorganise items in the home to help conserve energy. For example, in the kitchen, positioning the kettle near the sink and the fridge, and keeping cups near the kettle, means all items for making a hot drink are easily accessible from one place.

Reflection Point 5.1   Environment: The bedroom

Think about the layout of your bedroom, its contents and your routine in the morning. How could you reorganise your bedroom to make it easier to get dressed in the morning?

Comprehensive training in enabling techniques and working with a clear reablement plan is essential to empower support workers to work with service users to achieve their outcomes. The support worker role in reablement services will continue to evolve. The Care Council for Wales commissioned a report on the 'care at home' workforce. A number of local authorities in Wales reported that they were developing a health and social care support role. The descriptions of this role in the different areas include undertaking nursing, therapy and social care roles; and working across short-term and long-term services, including reablement (Llewellyn et al. 2010). One district describes the support worker having an outcomes-based approach following service users through different services. While this role appears beneficial for service users, supervision and training would need to be robust to enable support workers to work across diverse areas of practice. Reablement is an approach to service users that involves person-centredness and teamworking to achieve goals that motivate them, as well as developing a set of skills to help achieve them.

Scenario 5.1   Spending time with Beth

An example of person-centred working in a reablement service

Beth was referred to a reablement service as she was finding it more difficult to prepare food and it was reported that she had lost weight.

Jan, an OT, visited Beth to complete an assessment and agree goals with Beth. During her assessment Beth explained to Jan that as she had arthritis, particularly

▶

◄

affecting her hands, she was finding it more difficult to get things out of the oven. She said that she enjoyed cooking but had not felt like cooking and had lost her appetite since her husband died four months ago. Beth said that her husband used to help open cans and lift dishes out of the oven. She has a microwave in her bungalow but stated that the microwave had been bought for her and she has never used it. Beth told Jan that she was not keen on having hot meals delivered or on having support workers visit her and make her a meal. She knew, however, that she had been finding cooking too difficult and it was now affecting her quality of life.

Jan described the approach of the reablement team as a team that would support Beth to be able to do the things she wanted to do. Beth said that cooking had been important for her and that she would like to cook again. Jan and Beth agreed a goal for her reablement plan so that she would be able to prepare snacks and heat meals independently.

It was important that the support workers had a friendly and encouraging approach with Beth as she had said that she was not keen on having people in her house. After careful consideration and discussion with her, it was decided that Beth would have a specific support worker for each session rather than different people coming to her every day. The service had capacity to do this. Fran, the support worker, discussed meals with Beth and started by visiting her every lunch time. She provided verbal prompts and support to enable Beth to heat up frozen meals, to help her gain confidence in using her microwave. Fran demonstrated the controls on the microwave. To simplify the process, she marked the frozen meal boxes with the cooking time needed to heat up the meal in the microwave. After each visit Fran recorded in Beth's notes what Beth had achieved and/or been supported with. For example, she recorded that Beth had remembered the steps of removing the lid of the frozen meal and set the correct heat and time on the microwave, but had asked Fran to get the meal out of the microwave.

Fran quickly established that Beth was not keen on getting the meal out of the microwave as she was worried that she would drop it or burn herself. The meal needed to be carried to the adjacent worktop. Fran discussed this with Beth and suggested that the microwave could be moved to another area of the kitchen where there was more room in front of the microwave. The microwave was moved and Beth was able to lift her meal the short distance from her microwave to the worktop.

As Beth's confidence in heating up meals, and motivation to eat increased, Fran started to work with Beth on cooking simple meals from scratch in the microwave such as baked potatoes. They then moved onto a one-minute quiche in a mug. Fran had found a website that enables healthy cooking from scratch in a microwave, from macaroni cheese to a cup of coffee cake. Beth was delighted but as she had grown to trust Fran she told her that she missed eating with people. So Fran accompanied Beth to a local lunch club on two occasions until she felt confident enough to go alone. Beth arranged to attend the lunch club once a week and within four weeks Beth was making her own meals and no longer required support from the reablement service. In addition, and at a later date following a review, it transpired that Beth met another woman of a similar age at the club. They no longer attended but every week one of them would take a taxi to the other's home and they would cook a meal and eat it together.

Learning and development

As with all roles in the reablement service, support workers need to undertake regular training to maintain their ability to do their job. Providing a 'quality' service relies in part on the knowledge, skills and capabilities of the workforce delivering the service. Support workers are the team members working on a day-to-day basis with service users. Maintaining and developing their skills is important in order to deliver the best possible service to the service user.

Learning and development activities range from mandatory training to informal learning activities undertaken by the individual. These types of learning activities will be explored later in the chapter. **Continuing professional development (CPD)** is the term often used to categorise the learning and development activities undertaken by registered health and social care professionals (like OTs, PTs and social workers) in order to maintain their registration. These professionals are regulated by bodies such as the Health and Care Professions Councils. The regulator stipulates what CPD (learning and development activities) a registrant should complete and monitors this through an audit process, where registrants sign each time they renew their registration and can be selected to show evidence on how they have met the standards of CPD.

Currently, support workers working in health and social care do not have to be registered. The Royal College of Nursing (RCN) writes that CPD 'is fundamental to the development of all health and social care practitioners and is the mechanism through which high quality patient and client care is identified, maintained and developed' (RCN 2007, p. 2). CPD has at its core the concept of developing oneself and one's practice through lifelong learning, including both experiential learning, increased understanding of theoretical concepts and reflection on the relationship between the two to develop greater competency in practice. Thinking about CPD is just as relevant therefore for support workers, as undertaking activities linked to professional development will help support workers to develop knowledge, skills and capabilities which not only give personal satisfaction – with the individual knowing that they are giving the best possible service to clients – but may also provide evidence for consideration of career progression. For some support workers, CPD may be an opportunity to consider formal training to become a regulated health or social care practitioner in the future. With the advent of the recent Care Certificate (CQC 2015), it will be interesting to see how this will develop.

The Health and Social Care Act (DH 2008) established the Care Quality Commission as an independent regulatory body of health and social care services in the UK. Reablement is one of the services regulated by the Care Quality Commission. One of the areas the Care Quality Commission regulates is the recruitment and training of staff.

Regulation 22 of the Health and Social Care Act 2008 (Regulated Activities) Regulations 2010 states that:

> In order to safeguard the health, safety and welfare of service users, the registered person must take appropriate steps to ensure that, at all times, there are sufficient numbers of suitably qualified, skilled and experienced persons employed for the purposes of carrying on the regulated activity.

Reablement services are therefore expected to provide suitable induction, training, supervision and appraisal of staff. The Care Quality Commission expects employers of support workers to follow the 15 standards of the Care Certificate (CQC 2015). The Care Certificate is the minimum standard that should be undertaken as induction training for new support workers.

There is no standard specific training package for reablement services. The range and duration of induction and training for support workers is varied across organisations. In a study of reablement services in five different local authorities, induction periods for new support workers ranged from half a day to two weeks (Rabiee et al. 2009). Opportunity for training is a key factor in attracting and retaining support staff in social care (Skills for Care 2009). Some reablement services use external providers to provide their training for support staff (King et al. 2012). This has a cost attached to it and, as finances are reduced, services are considering different options for the delivery of services including training. This provides opportunities to consider different methods of delivering reablement training to find the most cost-effective quality option. The Social Care Institute for Excellence (SCIE) provides excellent free online modules for both managers and reablement workers, which are well worth a visit.

Mandatory training

Mandatory training is training that an employer identifies as essential training for an employee to do their job role. It covers training such as moving and handling and a food preparation certification. Often this training has to be undertaken during an induction phase of the roles and then updated in an annual cycle. Mandatory training will be a requirement for all staff and is not usually tailored to individual workers' needs.

Formal qualifications

Formal learning usually relates to undertaking a formal qualification. In the UK many local authorities recruit support workers with National Vocational Qualifications (NVQs) such as the NVQ 2 or NVQ 3 in care qualifications or support them to obtain this qualification (Nancarrow et al. 2005; Rabiee et al. 2009). The NVQ was replaced in 2010 by the Qualifications and Credit Framework (QCF) for England, Northern Ireland and Wales and in Scotland the Scottish Qualification and Credit Framework. The QCF offers qualifications made up of units of learning that have specific education credit. Learners complete units at their own pace and build up units of credit to gain an award, usually a certificate or diploma. The Health and Social Care Diploma is part of the CQF. The level 4 diploma in adult care (England) includes optional modules on developing and implementing reablement plans and on assistive technology [equipment] (Skills for Care 2015). Units of learning are also focused on the learner's workplace, and assessment is often linked to practice (work-based learning). In some services holding a formal qualification at a particular level is linked to career progression.

Competency-based qualifications, such as the NVQ and QCF units, present challenges to the service. The process of assessing support workers in a service user's home has been considered administratively problematic and ethical issues concerning confidentiality, privacy and personal dignity for service users have been raised (Bell 2001). However, **clinical supervision** and reflection on practice to plan future actions can follow on naturally from episodes of supervised care to demonstrate skills, competency and knowledge related to practice (Ball and Manwaring 2010).

Other learning activities

There are a range of other learning activities a support worker might engage in, for example a training workshop on a particular topic. These activities might be external to the service run by a national training organisation and often will have costs associated with them. Alternatively, other members of the team may organise internal training, sharing their own knowledge and skills. Team-based learning can be beneficial both for the individual but also to promote and support teamworking. Informal events such as journal clubs (where team members discuss a published article on a related topic) can also be helpful in sharing knowledge and experience.

Some reablement services have developed **competency** checklists for support workers and used role play and shadowing as training tools (Baker et al. 2001; Calderdale Council & Yorkshire and Humber Joint Improvement Partnership 2010). Silver Chain, a large provider of reablement services in Australia, has developed its own training programme manual (Silver Chain 2007). Wendy O'Connor, an OT in the UK, has developed useful training materials for reablement team members covering the ethos of reablement, activity analysis and agreeing outcomes. The material contains a number of practical activities for staff to try to introduce them to the difficulties experienced by some service users (O'Connor 2013).

The training and experience of OTs working across health and social care place them in an ideal position to facilitate training in reablement services. OTs are trained in rehabilitation techniques and enabling people to complete their daily occupations however their disabilities, age, difficulties or injury may affect them. Reablement is a service with a specific focus, working with service users with a variety of different disabilities and difficulties. Reablement services working specifically with people who have dementia and mental health problems are emerging. Many service users with dementia may currently be included in non-specialist reablement services. A review of dementia care both in community centres and in home care settings in Canada reported that 65% of staff felt that their prior knowledge and training were not sufficient to enable them to care for people with dementia (Jansen et al. 2009). Training in working with people with dementia and other long-term conditions aids the effectiveness of reablement services. Reablement staff have welcomed the input of OTs to give advice and increase the knowledge and skills of support staff (McLeod and Mair 2009; Latif 2011). Table 5.3 provides suggested topics to be included in reablement support worker training.

The opportunities and challenges of being a reablement support worker

The majority of support workers from traditional home care settings work part-time (Jorgensen et al. 2009). The role of a reablement support worker can fit flexibly around family commitments or part-time study. Reablement is typically a short-term service. This means that support workers need to establish rapport and a working relationship with service users quickly. This working relationship is often cited as the rewarding element of the job (King et al. 2012). The end of this short-term relationship can be difficult for service users who miss the social interaction with the support workers (Glendinning and Newbronner 2008). It can also be a challenge for support workers when they finish working with a service user. However, seeing a person reach a certain level of autonomy is a positive aspect of the support worker role and enables support workers to move on to enable others.

> *I enjoy more flexibility as a support worker, finding out about resources in the community for service users. (Reablement support worker)*

Table 5.3   Suggested training topics for reablement support workers

A move from a 'task-led' service to a person-centred, outcomes-based service	Communication and the development of respectful relationships to promote person-centred care. Practising good listening skills. Asking open and closed questions. Encouraging and motivating service users and managing expectations.
Team working	Understanding the roles of the different team members and when to refer to another member of the team.
Working in someone's home	Being respectful that you are in someone's home. The value of working in a service user's own environment and recognising that service users will have their own routines.
Importance of recording	How to record notes in the service user's home with sufficient information to enable the next support worker to work with the service user effectively. **Ineffective:** *'Beth undressed and supported to get into bed.'* **Effective:** *'Beth managed to remove most of her clothes. Support worker assisted to take Beth's socks off. Beth sat on edge of bed and support worker assisted to lift legs into bed as Beth stated she is tired today.'*
Physical disabilities and mental health problems and their effect on service users	Providing information and an overview of physical disabilities, mental health problems and learning disabilities and how these difficulties may affect the service user's ability to complete daily living activities.
Skills and techniques required for home care reablement	Skills in observation and encouragement. Use of activity analysis, backward chaining and energy conservation.
How equipment and adaptations support reablement	Demonstration and practice with different items of equipment that may adapt an activity to make it easier for service users.
Resources in the community	An overview of resources that service users may access in the community such as luncheon clubs, social groups and activity clubs.

Potential for support workers in the development of reablement services

The organisation Help the Aged coined the term 'social health' as essential to quality of life. This includes maintaining participation in interests, meeting friends and involvement in society (Harding 1997). Support with participating in social activities is not consistently included in reablement services (Bridges and James 2012). While support workers may wish to work in a holistic way meeting all the service user's outcomes, there is often a focus on personal care tasks in reablement services. Signposting people to other voluntary and statutory organisations is seen as a core element for reablement services (Glendinning and Newbronner 2008). Knowledge of local resources will enable reablement support workers to provide information to service users. Some service users may need more support than simple signposting. Reablement support workers can play a key role in supporting people to access other sources of social contact such as interest groups and befriending services as part of a reablement plan (see Chapter 3). For example, accompanying a service user, who continues to have difficulties cooking, to attend a local bowls club where they also have lunch together may lead to the service user making new friends alongside having a meal prepared for them. Supporting service users to increase their 'social health' in this way can reduce the need for ongoing support from social care services.

This chapter has considered the development of the support worker role and how support workers appreciate working with service users to support them to do the activities that are important to them. An overview of the equipment and techniques that may be used by reablement support workers in reablement services has been evaluated. The training and education needs of support workers have been considered and a suggested list of topics for reablement training of support workers suggested. The chapter concluded with the challenges and opportunities in developing the support worker role in reablement services.

Summary

> Reablement is a move from a 'doing to' approach to a 'doing with' person-centred approach.

> Reablement support workers work with service users to achieve their goals.

> Equipment can support people to become more independent.

> Activity analysis, backward chaining and energy conservation are all techniques that reablement support workers may use with service users.

> Training is essential for support workers to develop knowledge and skills in reablement.

> Working with people in a holistic way can be very rewarding for support workers.

> The addressing of social needs is a potential area for reablement support workers to develop but it may well be interesting and rewarding too.

Recommended reading

O'CONNOR, W. (2013) *Introduction to reablement: A work-based learning programme.* Hove: Pavilion Publishing and Media.

A useful e-learning module from the SCIE:
SCIE (SOCIAL CARE INSTITUTE FOR EXCELLENCE). (2013) *Reablement for care workers.* Available at: http://www.scie.org.uk/publications/elearning/reablement/ (Accessed 20 February 2015).

References

ALLEN, K. & GLASBY, J. (2010) The (multi-) billion dollar question: Embedding prevention and rehabilitation in English health and social care. *Journal of Integrated Care*, vol. 18, no. 4, 26–34.

BAKER, D. I., GOTTSCHALK, M., ENG, C., WEBER, S. & TINETTI, M. E. (2001) The design and implementation of a restorative care model for home care. *The Gerontologist*, vol. 41, no. 2, 257–263.

BALL, I. & MANWARING, G. (2010) *Making it work: A guidebook exploring work-based learning.* Gloucester: Quality Assurance Agency for Higher Education.

BARNES, P. A. & FROCK, A. H. (2003) The expanded role for rehabilitation in home care. *Home Health Care Management & Practice*, vol. 15, no. 4, 305–313.

BELL, L. (2001) Competence in home care. *Quality in Ageing*, vol. 2, no. 2, 13–20.

BORELL, L. (2008) Occupational therapy for older adults: Investments for progress. *British Journal of Occupational Therapy*, vol. 71, no. 11, 482–486.

BRIDGES, E. & JAMES, V. (2012) *Getting back on your feet: Reablement in Wales.* Cardiff: WRVS.

BUNNIN, A. (2011) *Understanding reablement.* London: Office for Public Management.

CALDERDALE COUNCIL & YORKSHIRE AND HUMBER JOINT IMPROVEMENT PARTNERSHIP. (2010) *Establishing best practice in reablement: 'People matter'.* Social Care Online. Available at: https://www.scie-socialcareonline.org.uk/establishing-best-practice-in-reablement-people-matter/r/a11G00000017x-H0IAI (Accessed 14 December 2017).

CARE SERVICES EFFICIENCY DELIVERY. (2007) *Homecare re-ablement workstream.* Discussion Document HRA 002. London: Department of Health.

CQC (CARE QUALITY COMMISSION). (2015) *CQC welcomes launch of the Care Certificate from April.* [Online]. http://www.cqc.org.uk/content/cqc-welcomes-launch-care-certificate-april. (Accessed 23 March 2017).

DH (DEPARTMENT OF HEALTH). (2007) *Putting people first. A shared vision and commitment to the transformation of Adult Social Care.* London: DH.

DH (DEPARTMENT OF HEALTH). (2008) *Health and Social Care Act.* London: HMSO.

DH (DEPARTMENT OF HEALTH). (2009) *Transforming Adult Social Care LAC (DH)*. London: DH.

DH (DEPARTMENT OF HEALTH). (2010) *A vision for adult social care: Capable communities and active citizens*. London: DH.

DH (DEPARTMENT OF HEALTH). (2014) *Care Act 2014*. London: DH.

DLF (DISABLED LIVING FOUNDATION). (2015) *Trusted assessor training*. Available at: http://www.dlf.org.uk/content/trusted-assessor-training (Accessed 24 February 2015).

DREILING, D. (2009) Energy Conservation. *Home Health Care Management and Practice*, vol. 22, no. 1, 26–33.

EBENSTEIN, H. (1998) From the world of practice. They were once like us: Learning from home care workers who care for the elderly. *Journal of Gerontological Social Work*, vol. 30, no. 3/4, 191–201.

GLENDINNING, C. & NEWBRONNER, E. (2008) The effectiveness of home care reablement – developing the evidence base. *Journal of Integrated Care*, vol. 16, no. 4, 32–39.

HARDING, T. (1997) *A life worth living: The independence and inclusion of older people*. London: Help the Aged.

HOCKING, C., MURPHY, J. & REED, K. (2011) Strategies older New Zealanders use to participate in day-to-day occupations. *British Journal of Occupational Therapy*, vol. 74, no. 11, 509–516.

JANSEN, L., FORBES, D. A., MARKLE-REID, M., HAWRANIK, P., KINGSTON, D., PEACOCK, S., HENDERSON, S. & LEIPERT, B. (2009) Formal care providers' perceptions of home- and community-based services: Informing dementia care quality. *Home Health Care Services Quarterly*, vol. 28, no. 1, 1–23.

JORGENSEN, D., PARSONS, M., REID, M. G., WEIDENBOHM, K., PARSONS, J. & JACOBS, S. (2009) The providers' profile of the disability support workforce in New Zealand. *Health and Social Care in the Community*, vol. 17, no. 4, 396–405.

KIELHOFNER, G. & FORSYTH, K. (2009) Activity Analysis. In E. A. S. Duncan (ed.) *Skills for practice in occupational therapy*. Edinburgh: Churchill Livingstone.

KING, A. I., PARSONS, M., ROBINSON, E. & JÖRGENSEN, D. (2012) Assessing the impact of a restorative home care service in New Zealand: A cluster randomised controlled trial. *Health & Social Care in the Community*, vol. 20, no. 4, 365–374.

LATIF, Z. (2011) *Cost benefit analysis of the Occupational Therapist's impact on reablement in Nottingham city*. Nottingham: Nottingham City Council.

LLEWELLYN, M., LONGLEY, M., FISK, M., BOUTALL, T., WALLACE, C. & ROBERTS, M. (2010) *Care at home: Challenges, possibilities and implications for the workforce in Wales*. Cardiff: Care Council for Wales.

MCLEOD, B. & MAIR, M. (2009) *Evaluation of City of Edinburgh council home care re-ablement service*. Edinburgh: Scottish Government Social Research.

NANCARROW, S. A., SHUTTLEWORTH, P., TONGUE, A. & BROWN, L. (2005) Support workers in intermediate care. *Health & Social Care in the Community*, vol. 13, no. 4, 338–344.

NEWBRONNER, E., BAXTER, M., CHAMBERLAIN, R., MADDISON, J., ARKSEY, H. & GLENDENNING, C. (2007) *Research into the longer term effects/impacts of re-ablement services.* London: Care Services Improvement Partnership/Care Services Efficiency Delivery Programme.

NORRIS, R. (2008) A reabling approach. *Commissioning News*, vol. 10, 8–9.

NORTHERN IRELAND ASSEMBLY. (2009) *Health and Social Care (Reform) Act (Northern Ireland) 2009.* Belfast: Northern Ireland Assembly.

O'CONNOR, W. (2013) *Introduction to re-ablement. A work-based learning programme.* Hove: Pavilion Publishing and Media.

OFFICE FOR PUBLIC MANAGEMENT. (2010) *Reablement: A guide for frontline staff.* London: Office for Public Management.

RABIEE, P. & GLENDINNING, C. (2011) Organisation and delivery of home care re-ablement: What makes a difference? *Health & Social Care in the Community*, vol. 19, no. 5, 495–503.

RABIEE, P., GLENDINNING, C., ARKSEY, H., BAXTER, K., JONES, K. C., FORDER, J. E. & CURTIS, L. A. (2009) *Investigating the longer term impact of home care re-ablement services: The organisation and content of homecare re-ablement services: Interim Report.* London: Department of Health/Care Services Efficiency Delivery.

RCN (ROYAL COLLEGE OF NURSING). (2007) *Joint Statement of Continuing Professional Development for Health and Social Care Practitioners.* London: RCN.

SCHREIBMAN, L. (1985) Backward chaining. In S. A. Bellack & M. Hersen (eds) *Dictionary of behavior therapy techniques.* New York: Pergamon Press.

SCIE (SOCIAL CARE INSTITUTE FOR EXCELLENCE). (2010) Personalisation briefing: implications for occupational therapists in social care. London: SCIE.

SCOTTISH PARLIAMENT. (2013) *Social Care (Self-directed Support) (Scotland) Act 2013.* Edinburgh: Scottish Parliament.

SILVER CHAIN. (2007) *Silver Chain's Home Independence Program (HIP). User manual.* Perth, Austalia: Silver Chain.

SINCLAIR, I., GIBBS, I. & HICKS, L. (2000) *The management and effectiveness of the home care services.* York: University of York Social Work Research and Development Unit.

SKILLS FOR CARE. (2009) *Attracting, retaining and developing staff in the adult social care sector in England: research briefing.* London: Skills for Care.

SKILLS FOR CARE. (2015) *Specification for level 4 Diploma in Adult Care (England).* [Online]. Available at: http://www.skillsforcare.org.uk/Documents/Learning-and-development/Qualifications/Level-4-diploma-in-health-and-social-care.pdf (Accessed 7 March 2017).

SOCIAL SERVICES IMPROVEMENT AGENCY. (2010) *A framework for reablement support worker training.* Cardiff: Social Services Improvement Agency.

WELSH ASSEMBLY GOVERNMENT. (2014) *Social Services and Well-being (Wales) Act 2014.* Cardiff: Welsh Assembly Government.

YU, D. S. F., LEE, D. T. F. & MAN, N. W. (2010) Fatigue among older people: A review of the research literature. *International Journal of Nursing Studies*, vol. 47, no. 2, 216–228.

6

Long-Term Conditions: Taking Control

E. Rose, S. Bintley-Bagot and L. Shorney

Chapter overview

This chapter will define long-term conditions (LTCs), exploring their prevalence and the potential for reablement within the context of current policy and guidelines. The impact of caring for someone with an LTC is considered and ways in which reablement can support informal carers are addressed.

What are long-term conditions (LTCs)?

LTCs are described as 'Chronic diseases, which current medical interventions can only control, not cure. The life of a person with a chronic condition is forever altered – there is no return to "normal"' (DH 2004, p. 3). Management is in the form of drugs alongside other treatment and interventions (Ross, Curry and Goodwin 2011). LTCs are insidious when they last longer than a year and service users may require ongoing care and support and, as Davies (2010) states, 'people with two or more LTCs are more likely to be obese, eat less healthily and smoke than people with one or none of these conditions' (p. 49).

There is now a global challenge caring for people with LTCs. In developing countries, the ageing population is growing due to exponential improvements in treatments and technological advances. The World Health Organization (WHO 2012) reports that health care systems worldwide are faced with the challenge of responding to high levels of population need, including chronic medical conditions such as diabetes, heart failure and mental illness, as evidenced in Box 6.1. Since 2005, UK national policy has placed more emphasis on the importance of managing and supporting people with LTCs in their own home, with the aim of reducing hospital admissions (DH

Acknowledgement to Louise Shorney, Senior Lecturer, University of Chester, for her contribution.

2005a, 2013, 2014a, 2015; IPPR 2014; DH). Promoting care closer to home, and empowering patients, service users and carers to make informed choices regarding their health and well-being, have added to these agendas.

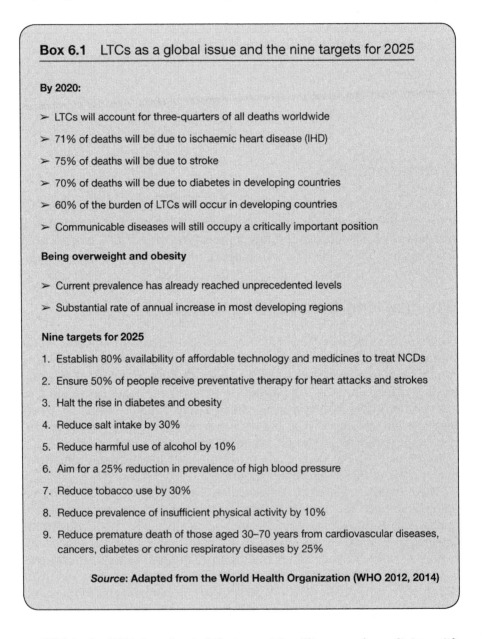

Box 6.1   LTCs as a global issue and the nine targets for 2025

By 2020:

➢ LTCs will account for three-quarters of all deaths worldwide

➢ 71% of deaths will be due to ischaemic heart disease (IHD)

➢ 75% of deaths will be due to stroke

➢ 70% of deaths will be due to diabetes in developing countries

➢ 60% of the burden of LTCs will occur in developing countries

➢ Communicable diseases will still occupy a critically important position

Being overweight and obesity

➢ Current prevalence has already reached unprecedented levels

➢ Substantial rate of annual increase in most developing regions

Nine targets for 2025

1. Establish 80% availability of affordable technology and medicines to treat NCDs

2. Ensure 50% of people receive preventative therapy for heart attacks and strokes

3. Halt the rise in diabetes and obesity

4. Reduce salt intake by 30%

5. Reduce harmful use of alcohol by 10%

6. Aim for a 25% reduction in prevalence of high blood pressure

7. Reduce tobacco use by 30%

8. Reduce prevalence of insufficient physical activity by 10%

9. Reduce premature death of those aged 30–70 years from cardiovascular diseases, cancers, diabetes or chronic respiratory diseases by 25%

Source: **Adapted from the World Health Organization (WHO 2012, 2014)**

Within the UK it is estimated that over 18 million people are living with LTCs requiring health and social care intervention. As intensive users of services, the impact of care on NHS and social care economies is profound and is expected to continue well into the future. The extent of this demand is illustrated in numerous publications. In Box 6.2 some useful ones are listed. These publications and websites outline the seriousness of LTCs in the UK and worldwide, but also their impact on individuals and how they can be managed.

Box 6.2 Publications outlining the impact and extent of LTCs on the public, UK health and social care services, and the economy

BRITISH MEDICAL ASSOCIATION. (2016) *Growing older in the UK: A series of expert-authored briefing papers on ageing and health*. Available at: http://www. bgs.org.uk/pdfs/2016bma_growing_older_in_uk.pdf (Accessed 20 January 2017).

COULTER, A., ROBERTS, S. & DIXON, A. (2013) Delivering better services for people with long-term conditions: Building the house of care. London: The King's Fund. Available at: http://www.kingsfund.org.uk/sites/files/kf/field/field_publication_file/ delivering-better-services-for-people-with-long-term-conditions.pdf (Accessed 2 May 2015).

WORLD HEALTH ORGANIZATION. (2014) *Together we can prevent and control the world's most common diseases*. Available at: http://www.who.int/nmh/ publications/ncd-infographic-2014.pdf?ua=1 (Accessed 2 February 2016).

It is estimated that caring for people with an LTC accounts for 70% (£7 out of every £10) of the money spent on health and social care in England, which means that 30% of the population account for 70% of the spend (Ross, Curry and Goodwin 2011; DH 2012a). One pound in every £8 spent on LTCs is linked to poor mental health and well-being (Naylor et al. 2012).

As a result of this increasing demand, health policy has attempted to refocus attention from a single service design to a more integrated service user-focused design. It is evident from the policy drivers (see Box 6.3) that health and social care organisations need to provide proactive, integrated and closer work between organisations and professionals. Essentially, this needs a person-centred approach to care which is closer to home, continuing the transformation in how care is delivered. This change in the caring paradigm can be challenging, but it is clear from the Five Year Forward View (DH 2014b) that there needs to be a new relationship with patients and communities, as well as new models of care. Patient 'activation' through reablement and empowerment is crucial to this paradigm shift.

Box 6.3   LTCs and the key policy drivers in the UK

➤ National Service Framework for Long Term Conditions (DH 2005a)

➤ Supporting people with long term conditions: Liberating the talents of nurses who care for people with long term conditions (DH 2005b)

➤ Supporting People with LTCs to Self Care (DH 2006)

➤ Long Term Conditions Compendium of Information (3rd edn) (DH 2012a)

➤ The NHS Mandate (DH 2012b)

➤ The NHS Outcomes Framework 2014/15: Domain 2 (DH 2013a)

➤ Transforming Primary Care (DH 2014a)

➤ Five Year Forward View (DH 2014b)

➤ Patients in control: Why people with long term conditions must be empowered (IPPR 2014)

➤ NHS Outcomes Framework 2016–2017 (DH 2016)

Delivering reablement services

The change in the delivery of care by reablement services has completely altered the philosophy of previous health care provision. The emphasis on reablement, rather than long-term care provision, where the service user can now have an element of choice and involvement in how and where support is needed to promote independence, is new and challenging, but also cost-effective (Glendinning et al. 2010; Wong 2010; Manthorpe 2011; Skelton 2013). This promotion of independence offers benefits to both the service user (see Chapters 4 and 7) and the wider economy and, arguably, to informal carers also.

Although reablement services are new and there are limited data on their benefits (Wilde and Glendinning 2012), initial reviews show that service user outcomes and satisfaction with the service remains high (Wong 2010; Manthorpe 2011; SCIE 2013; Skelton 2013). These services also meet key government targets (as identified in the key drivers in Box 6.3), which are essential to ensure that services are commissioned and continued in the future. For reablement services, preliminary studies have shown that targets such as delivering person-centred care, care that is closer to home, customising care to individual need and integrating reablement services with other care interventions can all be met very well (SCIE 2013).

Reablement services encourage interprofessional working, which is crucial to its success, but they also optimise the service user's potential for gaining independence throughout the process (see Chapter 4). Reablement teams can consist of occupational therapists (OTs), physiotherapists (PTs), nurses, dieticians, social workers, psychologists and podiatrists. However these services are made up, reablement support workers are their lifeline. They work very closely with professionals focusing on service users' overall health and well-being, and importantly in a reablement context, the chosen activities of daily living (ADL) they want to carry out independently. Their face-to-face contact time is often far greater on a one-to-one basis than that of the professionals. Individual clinicians have a skill base which is complex alongside advanced clinical reasoning, yet collectively will have considered care plans and integrated these into customised functional and goal-orientated tasks (Skelton 2013). These goal-orientated tasks can then extend to focus on specific tasks and skills required to complete **PADL or DADL** alongside hobbies, sports and other occupations. There has been an even greater shift when considering previous health care provision in juxtaposition with reablement philosophy. The requirement for home care support workers to move from a traditional formal 'hands-on' approach to one which is more 'hands-off' sits uncomfortably with many.

When home carers carry out reablement interventions this enables qualified health professionals to manage the more complex needs, assessing service users and providing objectives and tasks to be completed (Francis, Fisher and Rutter 2011; Wilde and Glendinning 2012). When support workers are involved in the delivery of reablement it means that the vast care needs of people across health and social care services can be addressed. Collectively reablement therapists and social care support workers are ideally placed to address this challenging increase in LTCs in society. (Rees 2014; Webster 2014). There is, however, a need for initial and ongoing training of support workers to equip them with the necessary skills, knowledge and attitudes to provide reablement rather than continuing the cycle of dependency (see Chapter 6).

Responses to Reablement

The majority of service users view reablement in a very positive light, seeing the benefit of improvement in functional ability, mobility and independence (Glendinning et al. 2010). Winkel, Langberg and Ejlersen (2015) found that even when people have been receiving care services previously, which is possibly the case for many people with LTCs, an improvement in ability to carry out ADL was still apparent after a

12-week reablement programme. It is therefore possible to draw the conclusion that those receiving home care services for any reason, including the management of an LTC, should not be excluded from reablement services.

There can, however, be varied responses to the reablement process. There can be different viewpoints, incentives, barriers, anxieties and fears that will have an impact on participation in reablement. Some of these barriers might be the fear of failing to improve or the need to show that there is an improvement between subsequent reablement interventions. There is also the fear of not being able to complete ADL on a day when the person's condition is worse – for example, when there is an exacerbation of pain or arthritic stiffness. This fear of failure may build up to a sense of loss, lack of security, lack of confidence, low mood and vulnerability. In addition, family support for the reablement process and viewpoint may be critical to its success.

There will inevitably be those service users who are fearful of the future and as a consequence take a more passive role within the process. Here the emphasis from the service user may be more directed as to how they are going 'to be made to get better' by the health care worker as opposed to how they are going 'to help themselves get better'. This emphasis drifts back to the historical model of health care and consequently society's perception of how health care should be delivered, a model where dependence on paid care is the norm. Added to this, some may have other genuine concerns about engaging in reablement. When successful it can impact on benefit entitlement. With the pressures of a government keen to reduce welfare benefits the incentive of reablement is paradoxically aligned with possible financial hardship for the person and their informal carer. As reablement is a fairly new and evolving service there is currently little research evidence to substantiate these responses. The media, however, have portrayed some of these disincentives in documentaries such as the Channel 4 series *Britain on benefits* and the BBC2 *Panorama* documentary 'Disabled or faking it' (broadcast 30 July 2012). Both documentaries have reviewed how people who are dependent on services may have a disincentive to progress, for example when offered a reablement service, for fear of losing benefits on which they depend.

The value of reablement

Reablement not only affects an individual, but also has a significant impact upon families, friends, carers and society as a whole. This section aims to explore the value of reablement from a variety of perspectives.

The individual

The aim of reablement is to help people to regain the ability to carry out their usual ADL. For someone with an LTC this may mean seeking 'new ways to do old things' (SCIE 2013a). The key to successful reablement is collaborative working. This is where a team of health and/or social care workers come together with the individual and their family to work towards agreed goals, acknowledging that every person brings equally valid knowledge and expertise from a professional or personal perspective (Davies 2000). The person being supported in reablement is at the centre of the plan, with co-partnership in developing meaningful, realistic and achievable goals (SCIE 2013a). If the person is willing and enthusiastic the process is more likely to succeed. Rather than a process involving an external locus of control (where professionals are seen as the only people able to bring about improvement), the service user should be enabled to have an internal drive towards achieving their objective/s (self-determination or motivation). This is why the service user needs involvement in setting their own goals and a trusting relationship with the reablement worker (see Chapter 7).

Following a period of reablement a positive outcome should mean more confidence in abilities with independent function that is 'good enough' for the individual. Remember that good enough to a person may have to be good enough for the home care support worker and professionals involved. For instance, the method of making a hot drink still involves an element of risk when the reablement service withdraws, but if the service user accepts this, making an informed choice, their autonomy may be respected, provided they are mentally competent (someone with dementia, for instance, may need alternative arrangements). However, facilitating an activity such as going to the pub may not be something that a therapist feels comfortable with in certain situations. This could be because of a person's ability to subsequently ingest alcohol safely as a result of medication, or to return safely home after social drinking, due to balance issues. Such concerns would require discussion and negotiation with the service user.

Reablement: Dementia

It is acknowledged that there is limited evidence to support the effectiveness of reablement for people with dementia, predominantly due to this client group being excluded from research (SCIE 2013b). However, in practice there are increasing numbers of practitioners who believe that reablement can be beneficial. SCIE (2013b) suggests that, when using a reablement approach with people with dementia, the goals are likely to be around 'preserving and encouraging a more functional state rather than achieving independence'. It is also suggested that reablement may focus on reducing social isolation, establishing routines and supporting the carers (SCIE 2013b). When encouraging social interaction, the role of the reablement practitioner will be to encourage the person to identify potential social situations they may enjoy and then support them in gaining access to their preferred activities or group situations. A focus may also be on exploring methods to remind the person about the social event or group. This will be different for each individual, for where some may respond to a calendar, others may require telephone prompts, for example. Establishing a routine with a person who has dementia is vital as it can help to keep him/her focused and may assist in embedding the activities into the long-term memory. The routine should include things that the individual has always done, for example reading the newspaper mid-morning or listening to a particular radio show. Other things to include could be medication reminders, toileting, bathing, personal grooming and leisure activities. Methods such as repetition (where the person does the same thing at the same time each day), charts and tick lists have been used to assist people in remembering what they need to do and when. A chart needs to be easily visible to prompt the person with dementia to follow it.

When working with people who have dementia it is important to emphasise the impact of the environment and how it can be adapted to enable individuals to function. Housing can be made 'dementia-friendly' when aspects such as lighting, acoustics, colour contrast and technology are incorporated (Dementia Services Development Centre 2017; NHS Choices 2015). During a reablement programme practitioners may wish to consider ways to support the person with dementia in navigating around the property. This would include labelling cupboards and drawers to remind the person of their content. The labels may be words, symbols or photographs depending on what works for the individual. Transparent doors on cupboards are often used so contents can be seen. Technology may be beneficial in supporting a person with dementia to function within the home environment, where items such as **pill dispensers** (an automated system which contains the required medication and is set to alarm at times when the medication is required), electronic diaries, automatic telephone reminders and **flood detectors** (which have sensors that trigger an audible alarm and can link to a system where a carer is alerted by telephone if a flood occurs), could all be used to maximize and prolong independence. This and other assistive devices are discussed in more depth in Chapter 8.

Practitioners must however consider the diagnosis and the impact of change. Often modern technologies can cause confusion, as people with dementia have difficulty learning new things and remembering how things work. It is therefore felt that traditional fittings are more appropriate, for example taps, bath plugs, toilet flushes. These familiar objects can be reassuring in a time of confusion (Dementia Services Development Centre 2017; NHS Choices 2015). However, Graff and colleagues (2006) found that the daily functioning of people with dementia improved following occupational therapy (OT) interventions despite the person's limited learning ability, and the effects were still present after 12 weeks; therefore, it is important to consider the stage of dementia and the likelihood of someone accepting new technologies as these will impact upon success. When working with a person with dementia it is generally advisable to avoid the implementation of major changes but rather encourage small, simple modifications than can make a clear difference (NHS Choices, 2015).

Student Activity 6.1 Reablement and the person with dementia

Highlight the key aspects that this section has taught you regarding reablement with a person who has dementia.

Reablement: Depression

Depression is a broad term used to describe a mental health condition which centres around severe low mood, often resulting in a loss of pleasure in most activities (NICE 2015; Leahy, Holland and McGinn 2012). If considered in the context of mental health, reablement might involve the person taking control and re-engaging in social and community life in a way that is satisfying and meaningful. Tew and colleagues (n.d.) reiterate this by stating that reablement within mental health may involve achieving positive outcomes in relation to:

➤ empowerment, choice and control

➤ social inclusion

➤ personal relationships

➤ mental and emotional well-being

The National Institute for Health and Care Excellence (NICE 2009) recommends 'mindfulness based cognitive therapy for people who are currently well but have had at least three episodes of depression' (NICE 2009, section 1.9.1.8 'Psychological interventions for relapse prevention'). This is an approach which reablement workers should be aware of in order to best support people with depression. **Mindfulness** encourages people to pay attention to the world around them, in particular, their own thoughts and feelings. It is about becoming more aware of the present moment, noticing all sensations – smells, sights, sounds, textures and tastes. The aim of this approach is not about trying to change or fix anything, but to enable an individual to see the present moment clearly. Focusing on both internal and external feelings and sensations can help to overcome the dominant negative thoughts within one's mind. By practising this, it is anticipated that the person with depression will start to notice when irrational thoughts are taking over and can start to rationalise them, understanding that the thoughts are not in control (NHS Choices 2016). Evidence shows that where mindfulness practice is taught across a series of weeks, stress levels are reduced and mood can be lifted (NHS Choices 2014). When adopting this approach, it is recommended that a specific time of day is selected to begin with when there is opportunity to pay attention to all sensations. A positive aspect of mindfulness is that it can be practised anywhere.

Cognitive behavioural approaches are also frequently used when working alongside a person with depression. These approaches aim to alter the way a person thinks about a situation to ultimately change the displayed behaviours. These changes can be supported by:

➢ Making a note of the key events occurring at the time
  - Are there any specific events which seem to occur in the lead-up to an episode of low mood?
➢ Noting how the person behaves at these times
  - Do you notice them becoming more withdrawn or isolated?
➢ Considering how you set goals with the person
  - Make sure they are realistic and achievable in order to engage and motivate the person. Maybe think about how they can be made more complex as the person progresses
➢ Identifying the activities that the person enjoys doing or has enjoyed in the past
  - Things which bring about feelings of pleasure or competence. These are the positive behaviours which are to be encouraged and can form part of a reward-based process
  - Encourage self-reward, recognising and acknowledging when s/he has demonstrated positive behaviours

> Encouraging social skills
  - Encourage positive behaviours towards others such as greeting people, complimenting others, being reliable, improving personal hygiene and appearance levels. These behaviours take effort for people with LTCs and disability, so positive encouragement helps to maintain motivation
> Developing problem-solving skills
  - Support someone to recognise a problem and source solutions, creating plans and identifying resources

(Leahy, Holland and McGinn 2012, p. 24)

It is widely reported that exercise and a healthy diet is beneficial to people who have depression. Being physically active can lift mood and lower stress levels. The release of endorphins can increase self-esteem while the activity itself can distract from negative thoughts as well as increase social interaction. Despite this, many people with depression lack interest in their own well-being, leading them to forgo an adequate diet (Leahy, Holland and McGinn 2012). Severe depression can result in poor self-maintenance, where normal personal hygiene and appearance levels are reduced (Leahy, Holland and McGinn 2012). This can then have a negative influence on social interactions and external rewards. A reablement programme could assist in re-establishing routine for the individual, educating and supporting a healthy diet and encouraging participation in physical activity. Family and friends hold the key to success for many people who have mental health support needs when re-establishing well-being and social participation. This emphasises the importance of informal carers, which will be explored later in the section titled 'The issues faced by informal carers and the importance of their involvement'.

Student Activity 6.2   Reablement and depression

Identify the key points that you have learned about reablement for a person who has depression.

Reablement: Respiratory disorders

Reablement teams often provide services for people who have the long-term respiratory condition of chronic obstructive pulmonary disorder (COPD). The scenario below provides insight into how someone with COPD could be supported.

Scenario 6.1   Chronic obstructive pulmonary disorder: Terry

Terry is 60 years old and has chronic obstructive pulmonary disorder (COPD). He has recently been discharged from hospital with a home oxygen supply. He has always lived alone and does not drive. Terry will be attending a pulmonary rehabilitation programme at the outpatient clinic. Upon discharge he will be dependent upon a neighbour providing meals and supporting him with self-care. Terry has always been a private man and is keen to maintain his independence, particularly regarding washing, dressing, shopping and cooking. He has therefore been referred to the reablement team.

Student Activity 6.3   Thinking about Terry

List the feelings that Terry might be experiencing:

_____   _____
_____   _____
_____   _____
_____   _____

Identify ways in which reablement might benefit Terry:

_____   _____
_____   _____
_____   _____
_____   _____

The reablement team set about to educate Terry about the pacing of activities and to encourage him to consider ways to conserve energy throughout the day, thus maintaining the ability to complete all his chosen tasks. Through the use of energy-conservation techniques, such as planning tasks ahead, allowing time for rest and relaxation, sitting when possible to carry out grooming and domestic tasks such as the washing-up, cooking and ironing, Terry managed to continue to live independently ('Occupation, activity and task' were explored in Chapter 1).

When considering cooking, Terry needs to be able to choose a meal, shop for the ingredients and then prepare it. In each of these stages there are many cognitive and physical activities that Terry needs to be able to achieve. For instance, he needs to have the stamina to walk to the supermarket, but he physically struggles to reach the closest shop due to becoming breathless while walking up the hill. A possible solution might be for him to order ingredients online, allowing him to remain in control of his shopping while 'conserving' his limited energy for other more enjoyable tasks. However, it is vital that Terry maintains levels of activity and is encouraged to participate in daily exercise, as maintaining a level of fitness leads to longer term gains. Using ambulatory oxygen and a rollator frame (a system where a small oxygen tank is attached to a walking frame on wheels) Terry was able to walk to an alternative shop, which although further away was along a flat route. (For people with COPD hills are more tiring than a greater distance with no incline.)

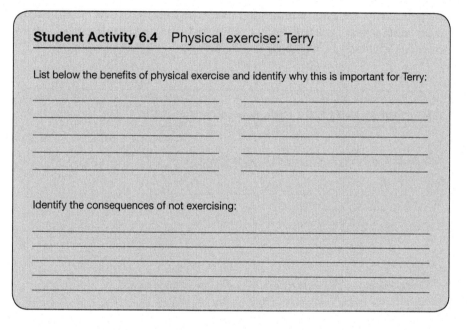

Student Activity 6.4   Physical exercise: Terry

List below the benefits of physical exercise and identify why this is important for Terry:

Identify the consequences of not exercising:

Activity analysis is implicit in the OT role, where each task is broken down into various components and then analysed in terms of the abilities required to carry out a task (Radomski and Latham 2008). **Chunking** is a technique where an activity is broken down into manageable 'chunks'. When considering cooking Terry was encouraged to select meals that could be prepared in stages. He prepares vegetables in the morning when his energy is at its height and then rests before cooking the meat rather than attempting to prepare the whole meal in one go. Another solution for Terry could be to purchase preprepared vegetables, thus saving energy.

The energy-conservation techniques utilised in this case also involve consideration of the environment. Terry was advised to rearrange his kitchen to enable easy access to the frequently used items, preventing excessive reaching, stretching or bending. Assistive aids were incorporated to reduce effort: a perching stool (a high stool with a sloping seat to aid functional posture while reducing the need to stand), a cooking basket (where the food is placed in the basket which in turn is lowered into a pan of water so preventing the need to lift the pan) and a kettle tipper (a device which a kettle fits into that can be lightly pushed to pour rather than lifted). A one-touch can opener (which only requires one press of a button to open tins) would also be helpful if Terry decides on using tinned food, and an electric whisk or food processor might be useful for other aspects of food preparation. Terry was encouraged to leave the washing-up to dry on a rack rather than use energy drying up. These methods enable new ways for him to continue to manage his own life independently. Chapter 5 reminded us of the importance of environmental considerations and this aspect is taken further when discussing technological advances in reablement (Chapter 8).

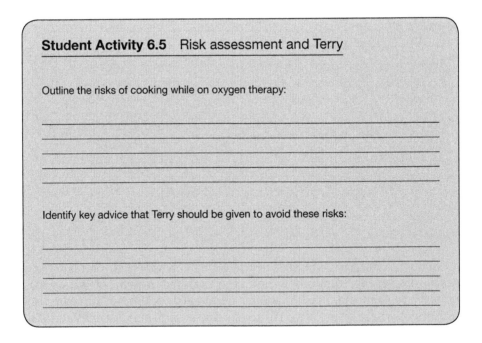

Student Activity 6.5   Risk assessment and Terry

Outline the risks of cooking while on oxygen therapy:

_____

_____

_____

_____

_____

Identify key advice that Terry should be given to avoid these risks:

_____

_____

_____

_____

_____

In order to maintain levels of self-care Terry was taught techniques to pace himself and reduce energy expenditure. A shower board, which is placed across the top of the bath creating a safe surface to sit on, was issued enabling him to rest while showering. Drying himself was always an activity that Terry found exhausting so he was encouraged to wrap himself in a towelling robe rather than physically drying himself. The reablement support worker worked with Terry to practise new dressing techniques to avoid the need for bending. *Bending is difficult for people with COPD as it reduces the space in the thoracic cavity making it difficult to breathe.* Terry was advised to sit down while dressing and to use small aids such as elastic shoe laces, a long-handled shoe horn and a sock aid.

Student Activity 6.6   Living with COPD

List below the key points that you have learned from this case study of reablement with a person who lives with chronic obstructive pulmonary disease (COPD):

_____
_____
_____
_____
_____

Clearly, the outcome of successful reablement leads to a reduction in visitors throughout the day. It is often no longer necessary for friends and family to call in to check on an individual, or help him/her. For some, this is a positive element, but for others this could lead to a sense of social isolation.

Student Activity 6.7   Rheumatoid arthritis and Grace

You have been working with 82-year-old Grace for the past six weeks following a flare-up of her rheumatoid arthritis. She lives alone and does not have any close family. Her neighbour, Helen, was her only friend, but Helen died a year ago.

You have used a reablement approach with Grace which has proved successful as she is now fully independent again. She looked forward to your visits and has really enjoyed your conversations but now it is time for you to discharge her from your service.

How might Grace be feeling?

_____
_____
_____
_____
                                                                ▶

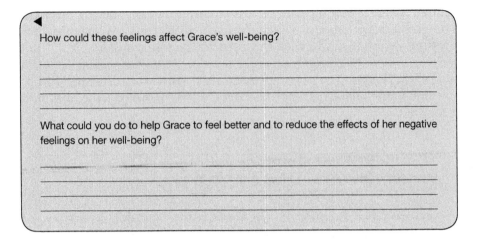

How could these feelings affect Grace's well-being?

_____

_____

_____

_____

What could you do to help Grace to feel better and to reduce the effects of her negative feelings on her well-being?

_____

_____

_____

_____

If the reablement worker is the only social contact a person has had when the process comes to an end the company and interaction may be sorely missed. A reduction in care hours for isolated people could lower their sense of well-being (Francis, Fisher and Rutter 2011). It is important to know whether the individual wants company and interaction so that social activities can be incorporated into a support plan, perhaps by accessing local community services and voluntary organisations. These do not have to be traditional day services for older people but ones organised by voluntary services such as Age UK, the University of the Third Age or classes in floristry or computing. If social welfare is not considered and the person becomes lonely and isolated, the motivation to continue using the skills developed through reablement could be compromised and therefore the person's health and well-being could decline. This is such an important aspect but quite often it is not adequately addressed.

Family, friends and carers

The Social Care Institute for Excellence (SCIE 2012) highlights that many families find the concept of reablement difficult as it is relatively new and they can feel uncomfortable relinquishing their care role. There still remains an expectation for people to be 'cared for' by their relatives and indeed statistics support this. England alone has in excess of 6 million informal carers (Schaffer 2013) which relieves the economy of a significant burden as it is estimated that, were each of these individuals paid a salary, it would amount to approximately £15,000 plus. In 2011, unpaid informal care was estimated at a value to society of £119 billion (NHS

Information Centre and Social Care Team 2010). In addition to this, there is further cost to carers including fatigue, isolation, exacerbation of existing conditions and the development of new ones. Additionally, employed informal carers lost working hours, and sometimes having to cease work is a significant issue, particularly for partners, who make up the majority of informal carers.

When reablement is in progress it is often challenging for informal carers, as they then have to stand back while someone struggles. This can generate feelings of anger or distress. It is often associated with guilt, especially if the family have been struggling alone for a long time. It is not uncommon for stress and fatigue of informal carers to negatively affect their relationship with the service user. Carers may be concerned about the risks involved in this approach so positive risk taking, the balance between risk and building independence, should be discussed (SCIE 2013b). Another often overlooked dimension is the change in relationship between a once independent couple to one where attendance to a partner's personal care such as bathing and incontinence makes up their everyday life. This is a particularly complex aspect of the care continuum. It is difficult to consider your partner romantically, let alone as a sexual being, in these situations. The effects on the self-concept of both partners, their expression of sexuality and the effects it may have on the relationship can be profound. So personal independence, and where necessary formal support, should be the goal of care to minimise feelings of loss of masculinity or femininity for the person and their partner, or feelings of asexuality, with loss of self-worth. Consider Scenario 6.2.

Scenario 6.2   Stroke and intimacy

Medical history

Mr Finson had a **haemorrhagic stroke** (caused by venous malformation) five years ago, resulting in limitations to movement in his left arm and **hemianopia**. Another problematic outcome of the stroke is **dysphagia** which predominantly causes him difficulties with swallowing. A speech and language therapist worked with him when he was in hospital to find safer strategies when eating, alongside exercises to improve his swallowing. He has a specific diet to help with this. Mr Finson suffers particularly with chronic constipation resulting in very unpleasant and painful haemorrhoids. This bothers him more than anything. He is not overweight.

Mrs Finson had a cardiac arrest about seven years ago and has some arthritis in her hands. Aside from this she is quite active, shopping locally with a trolley, and loves cooking for her husband.

▶

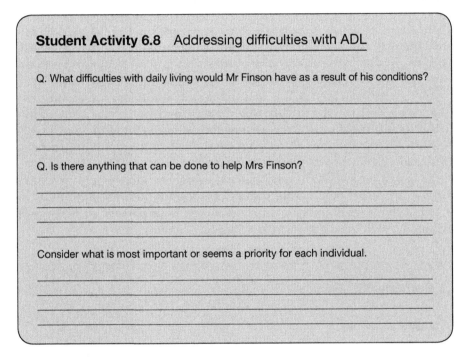

◀

Reason for reablement intervention

Mr and Mrs Finson, who are now 80 and 76 respectively, married in their 50s. They had a relationship in their 20s but for one reason or another had children with different partners. Approximately 30 years ago Mr Finson got in touch with his first love again. The couple are clearly devoted to each other but since Mrs Finson has had to assist her husband with his personal care, they are no longer intimate. She expresses this quite naturally to the OT and later on it transpires that she had also expressed her concerns to the district nurse involved.

Student Activity 6.8   Addressing difficulties with ADL

Q. What difficulties with daily living would Mr Finson have as a result of his conditions?

_____
_____
_____
_____

Q. Is there anything that can be done to help Mrs Finson?

_____
_____
_____
_____

Consider what is most important or seems a priority for each individual.

_____
_____
_____
_____

Discussion and reflection on Scenario 6.2

To the reablement team the issues were evident from the outset but they set out to discuss first what the couple wanted to achieve. The plan was immediately clear for Mr and Mrs Finson. It would meet both their needs as carer and service user. In partnership with a PT, the OT and nurse set about facilitating Mr Finson to self-care. They worked out different methods and techniques with him and provided some assistive aids. This included working out the best way for him to use a long-handled sponge and to transfer on and off safely from a drop-down shower seat with arm rests. This was fitted in the couple's walk-in shower room. An increase in contrast of colour and shades was added throughout the room using halogen lighters and some bright stickers to the existing toilet frame and areas around the walk-in shower (in particular on the drop-down rails). Some Dycem matting was also provided. Mr Finson's plate already included a guard but it often slid around on the table, so this was a simple solution. Overall, however, he was most pleased with his new-found ability to apply his suppositories while lying on the bed on his left side. It was not easy and it took several different approaches, but at the end of five weeks Mr Finson was able to wash himself and apply medicated suppositories and the difference was evident. There was no need for anything else because even though Mrs Finson took some time getting meals ready, she did this gladly and would not have it any other way – despite offers for formal care. The reablement support workers discussed some energy-conservation techniques with her. Mrs Finson found this useful as well as the kettle tipper and perching stool they provided for use in the kitchen. She declined a four-wheeled trolley. It was clear following a review a week later that their relationship had regained the intimacy that was lost temporarily. Co-working, patience and understanding made a great difference to this couple's life, and those involved (the PT, OT, nurse and reablement support workers) gained great satisfaction in the process and joint working to the positive conclusion.

Reflection Point 6.1   Helping to make reablement interventions successful: The importance of co-working and communication

This scenario emphasises the need for practitioners to explain the concept of reablement clearly to all involved, reassuring them that, although the aim is to restore independence, it is also about dignity. Families are an important part of the success of reablement, encouraging a round-the-clock approach to using new skills. Communication and a shared approach between the practitioner, the individual and those supporting the individual are therefore vital. Ensuring that the individual and his/her family form part of the team, from the start of the process to its conclusion, will assist in developing a mutual understanding of the reablement philosophy and ultimately lead to the independence of the service user.

The issues faced by informal carers and the importance of their involvement

When someone is struggling at home it is often family or friends who are the first port of call for help. This can be a source of frustration for both parties as it interrupts daily routines and can be invasive. For example, flare-ups of rheumatoid arthritis can appear with no obvious trigger and no particular pattern (Arthritis Research UK 2011). The unpredictable manner of this LTC makes it very difficult to plan ahead. It may be that the individual is independent for long periods of time, so not requiring any assistance, but during a flare-up the pain experienced may be such that the individual is unable to manage many daily activities. It is during this time that family or friends may be called upon. As it is difficult to predict when this support is needed, family and friends may have to make major adjustments to their daily lives in order to be available, such as taking paid holidays from work. This is frustrating and can make the individual feel guilty for asking for help.

The dynamics and roles in relationships naturally change as someone moves from being a daughter/son/friend/parent to being a carer. Reablement aims to reduce the need for support and care from friends and family and lessen the strain on family relationships (SCIE 2012). For some, this is a positive element as it means that they can resume their normal relationship. Rather than being a carer, the visits become social again instead of being focused around physical support. Successful reablement can lead to a healthy balance of caring and paid work along with other responsibilities. If, following the reablement process, a person still requires some form of care from family members, the carer is likely to be protected under the Equality Act (HM Government 2010) by association with a disabled person. This gives them the right to request flexible working in order to balance caring and paid work. Some informal carers have reported that being involved in reablement improves their confidence in their own caring abilities and responsibilities (Francis, Fisher and Rutter 2011).

Conversely, some informal carers may find the reduction in caring responsibilities difficult to manage. If this role had been a large part of their life they may experience significant identity change when this is no longer required. It is important to support carers through this transition by recognising that, although it could provide the opportunity for much needed rest, it can also leave them with a lot of time to fill (SCIE 2012). Reiterating the value of their ongoing support could assist with this transition. Families play a vital role in the long-term success of reablement by continuing to encourage the use of newly developed skills, thus maintaining confidence and motivation (SCIE 2012). This may be a different approach than the carer is used to as it will require them to stand back and give the person time, encouragement and space to practise doing things independently, rather than physically stepping in to help. Carers need to feel confident to be able to provide positive feedback to the individual and to assist in maintaining the motivation to achieve. They can do this by highlighting how well the individual is doing and reminding him/her of the long-term goals at times when s/he may feel like giving up. It is vital that carers understand their position in the reablement approach so that they are able to verbally support rather than through physical means. By emphasising the importance of this role, practitioners will be aiding the transition by reducing "hands-on care" while still maintaining a supportive and encouraging role for the informal carer.

Being looked after by informal carers can bring security and close support – something quite distinct from interventions carried out by paid staff (formal carers). This informal care is far more cost-efficient in the long term than numerous different services being brought to the home or provided in the community (Glendinning et al. 2010). However, many informal carers can suffer from exhaustion, stress and depression as well as social isolation, as caring takes its toll. It is also well known that many existing conditions are exacerbated or new ones develop as a result of physiological stress. Welfare benefits, such as disability living allowance, personal independence payment and attendance allowance, are given to the family member to cover the costs of their care and additional needs (Age UK 2014). The 'debt', however, for the informal carer is often great. So reablement can provide family members with regular financial support but this can pose problems when reablement interventions are withdrawn. This is because informal carers can then go back very easily to 'doing for' rather than 'doing less'. This is counterproductive and often occurs when carers have not been included in the service user's reablement care plan. Involving the service user's family and friends is supportive in the long term. They can offer some security and help improve confidence levels and reduce the fear of uncertainty, anxiety and isolation (Skelton 2013). When reablement interventions withdraw, the informal carer can continue to support the person with some tasks. On the other hand, they will have new knowledge and understanding of when and how to stand back and support the person to carry out daily activities independently. Have a look now at Scenario 6.3 and see whether you can describe and explain some of the issues that might occur for Mary, a 72-year-old widowed woman who lives alone.

Scenario 6.3   Hemiplegia and Mary

Background

Mary is 72. She was widowed 18 months ago but has been managing very well since. She lives alone in a semi-detached bungalow with a small garden. Her daughter, Jane, visits most weeks, helping with shopping or cleaning. Mary is very much an 'on the go' person, rarely sits down, enjoys a good network of friends and often has day trips out with Jane.

▶

◄

Event

Mary was doing some gardening at home when she had a cerebrovascular accident (CVA, or stroke). This resulted in an emergency admission to hospital where she was made medically stable. The CVA caused Mary to have left-sided **hemiplegia (paralysis of one side of the body)**.

Student Activity 6.9   Understanding Mary and her situation

Describe how Mary may be feeling at this time and the thoughts she may be having:

_____
_____
_____

Outline how you would expect Mary to progress while in hospital.

_____
_____
_____

What difficulties might Mary have in terms of her health and her ability to care for herself independently?

_____
_____
_____

How might this episode of illness and hospital admission affect Mary's social circumstances?

_____
_____
_____

Rehabilitation (inpatient)

During her time as an inpatient Mary received physiotherapy and OT, which led to her being able to get around with a walking stick, and transfer on and off her chair, bed and toilet independently. After two weeks she was desperate to return home but was still unable to wash and dress herself or prepare a meal. Seeing how distressed her mother was becoming, Jane offered to move in with her to care for her in order to speed up her discharge from hospital. This meant that Jane's husband was left to run the household, supporting their teenage sons.

Student Activity 6.10   The dual nature, and need on occasion, for combining 'doing for' with 'doing for self'

Describe how Mary may be feeling at this point in time and what her concerns might be:

Consider the possible effects on Jane and her family – what might their thoughts and feelings be?

Outline how you would expect Mary to progress on returning home to be cared for by her daughter Jane.

On discussion the OT raised concerns about the arrangement due to the potential stress that this situation could have on the mother–daughter relationship between Mary and Jane, and also the change in dynamics for Jane, her husband and their sons. Aware that most progress is made in the weeks immediately following the stroke, the OT recommended Mary for a reablement programme while Jane was living with her.

Student Activity 6.11   Reablement, relevant approaches and the impact on Mary's life

Describe ways in which Mary's health and well-being could be improved within a reablement programme:

Outline the most effective interventions/plans/approaches for enabling Mary to gain maximum independence – include Jane in your assessment.

▶

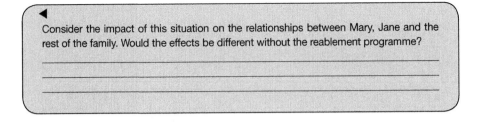

Consider the impact of this situation on the relationships between Mary, Jane and the rest of the family. Would the effects be different without the reablement programme?

_____

_____

_____

Reablement

A reablement programme was set in place with daily visits from a support worker who continued to work with Mary on personal care. Mary was provided with a stool specifically designed for use within the shower (after an assessment to show that there was adequate space within the cubicle) and grab rails were put in place to enable a safe transfer into and out of the shower. Small aids such as long-handled sponges and combs were trialled to enable Mary to manage her own personal hygiene and grooming. The reablement support worker demonstrated and practised dressing techniques with Mary which led to her dressing independently using a **helping hand, dressing stick** (which is a stick with a hook on the end) **and sock aid** (an item specifically designed to assist someone to put on their socks without the need to bend). The reablement support worker took time to establish the type of meals that Mary enjoyed and then worked alongside her to establish new ways to prepare these meals. Items such as a **spike board** (where items to be chopped are held in place by the spikes, meaning they can be chopped using only one hand), a **spreader board** (which is a board with raised edges at the corners which prevents bread from slipping when being buttered) and a one-handed tin opener were adopted to enable Mary to be independent.

After five weeks of reablement Mary was independent in washing, dressing and meal preparation. This gave her a sense of self-efficacy and self-esteem which meant that she was willing to go out with friends again. She was no longer dependent on Jane for any more than she had been prior to the CVA and Jane was able to return home.

Student Activity 6.12 Cognitive reframing for Mary

Consider Mary's feelings when Jane returns to her own home. Identify not only negative thoughts and feelings, but also the positive ones. See if you can then reframe (**cognitive reframing**) the difficult ones:

_____

_____

_____

▶

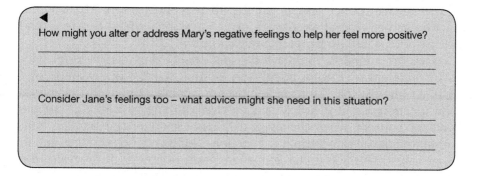

How might you alter or address Mary's negative feelings to help her feel more positive?

Consider Jane's feelings too – what advice might she need in this situation?

Societal perspectives

There are many aspects of society which depend greatly upon the con-tributions of a voluntary workforce, with the 'health and social work' employment category responsible for employing 60% of all volunteers in the UK in 2013 (Skills – Third Sector 2015). The employees within the voluntary sector tend to be older than those in the private and public sec-tors, with almost 40% being aged 50 or above (Skills – Third Sector 2015). Without these volunteers providing services and support to other mem-bers of society, the social care cost would amount to at least £87 billion per year. In 2007/08 local authorities spent £8.8 billion on personal social care for older people (SafeguardingUK 2014). As the age of the popula-tion increases, the demand on these services rises. If the cost of such services increases at the same rate as the population, it will almost dou-ble by 2026. It is therefore important to maintain the independence of people as they approach retirement and beyond, as without this group of volunteers providing care services publicly funded resources will be required. Research evidence shows that reablement improves independ-ence, prolongs ability to live at home and removes or reduces the need for commissioned care homes (Francis, Fisher and Rutter 2011).

In comparing reablement to conventional home care it is found that reablement improves physical functioning and reduces the needs for ongoing services. One study showed that up to 62% of people no longer required services after a 6–12-week reablement period compared with 8% of the control group (SafeguardingUK 2014). It is nonetheless evident that reablement services have a higher initial cost than traditional care packages (Glendinning et al. 2010). It can be argued that this is due to training needs, closer supervision of home care support workers and more responsive flexible visits. However, evidence shows that the initial cost is offset in the long term by the reduction in longer term social care needs (Francis, Fisher and Rutter 2011). Gerald Pilkington (previous national lead for home care reablement in the Department for Health) noted that if the average council adopts reablement they should save 220,000 contact hours per year, at an average of £15 per hour, which creates a total saving of £3.3 million per year (SafeguardingUK 2013).

LTCs are complex, multifactorial and challenging. Service users with LTCs represent a growing population in the UK who ideally are treated with an interdisciplinary team approach to promote safety, independence and functional ability. Reablement services can engage with this population and concept; when effectively delivered they provide a seamless transition from acute care settings to functional independence at home, and in some cases prevent hospital admissions from occurring. Early evaluation shows that such services benefit the social care economy and demonstrate a high acceptance and satisfaction to service users and families. Reablement for LTCs has shown it can meet government policy by providing localised, customised care by a range of health care professionals and home care support workers throughout the variable course of the condition.

Summary

➤ Long-term conditions (LTCs) are complex conditions.

➤ Reablement is effective for both long-term physical and mental health conditions.

➤ There is a growing population of those with LTCs that is affecting society.

➤ Government policy is changing to support this growth.

➤ Reablement is a rapidly growing service which aims to cease or reduce formal care.

➤ The service can be useful as a preventative mechanism.

➤ Interprofessional working is crucial to the success of reablement.

➤ Involvement of families alongside the service user, support workers and professionals is important.

➤ Consideration must be given to the impact that reduced social contact can have on an individual.

Recommended reading

GLENDINNING, C., JONES, K., BAXTER, K., RABIEE, P., CURTIS, L., WILDE, A., ARKSEY, H. & FORDER, J. (2010) *Home Care Re-ablement Services: Investigating the longer-term impacts (prospective longitudinal study)*. York: Social Policy

▶

◀

Research Unit, University of York. Available at: http://www.york.ac.uk/inst/spru/research/pdf/Reablement.pdf

FRANCIS, J., FISHER, M. & RUTTER, D. (2011) *Reablement: A cost-effective route to better outcomes*, London: SCIE.

MANTHORPE, J. (2011) *Benefits of home care reablement in the long term*. Community Care. Available at: http://www.communitycare.co.uk/2011/10/06/benefits-of-home-care-reablement-in-the-long-term/

SCIE (SOCIAL CARE INSTITUTE FOR EXCELLENCE) (2013a) *Maximising the potential of reablement*. SCIE guide 49. London: Author. Available at: http://www.scie.org.uk/publications/guides/guide49/

TEW, J., PLUMMIDGE, G., NICHOLLS, V. & CLARKE, H. (n. d). *Whole family approaches to reablement in mental health: Scoping current practice*. Birmingham: University of Birmingham.

WILDE, A. & GLENDINNING, C. (2012) 'If they're helping me then how can I be independent?' The perceptions and experience of users of home-care re-ablement services. *Health & Social Care in the Community*, vol. 20, no. 6, 583–590.

WINKEL, A., LANGBERG, H. & EJLERSEN, E. (2015) Reablement in a community setting. *Disability and Rehabilitation*, vol. 37, no. 15, 1347–1352.

References

AGE UK. (2014) *Love later life; Money matters*. Available at: http://www.ageuk.org.uk/money-matters/claiming-benefits/carers-allowance/ (Accessed 6 October 2014).

ARTHRITIS RESEARCH UK. (2011) *Rheumatoid Arthritis Handbook*. Available at: https://www.arthritisresearchuk.org/arthritis-information/conditions/rheumatoid-arthritis/self-help/managing-a-flare-up.aspx (Accessed 12 December 2017).

BICKLEY, L., SZILAGYI, P. & BATES, B. (2009) Bates' guide to physical examination and history taking. Philadelphia, PA: Wolters Kluwer Health/Lippincott Williams & Wilkins.

DAVIES, C. (2000) Getting health professionals to work together. *British Medical Journal,* vol. 320, no. 7241, 1021–1022.

DAVIES, N. J. (2010) Improving self-management for patients with long-term conditions. *Nursing Standard,* vol. 24, no. 25, 49–56.

DEMENTIA SERVICES DEVELOPMENT CENTRE. (2017) *Good practice in design for dementia and sight loss*. Available at: http://dementia.stir.ac.uk/design/good-practice-design-dementia-and-sight-loss (Accessed 2 December 2017).

DH (DEPARTMENT OF HEALTH). (2004) Chronic disease management: A compendium of information. Available at: http://www.natpact.info/uploads/Chronic%20Care%20Compendium.pdf (Accessed 2 December 2017).

DH (DEPARTMENT OF HEALTH). (2005a) National service framework: long term conditions. Available at: https://www.gov.uk/government/publications/quality-standards-for-supporting-people-with-long-term-conditions (Accessed 2 December 2017).

DH (DEPARTMENT OF HEALTH). (2005b) *Liberating the talents of nurses who care for people with long term conditions.* Available at: http://webarchive. nationalarchives.gov.uk/+/www.dh.gov.uk/en/Publicationsandstatistics/ Publications/PublicationsPolicyandGuidance/DH_4102469 (Accessed 2 December 2017).

DH (DEPARTMENT OF HEALTH). (2006) *Supporting people with long term conditions to … Self care. A guide to developing good policies and practice.* Available at: http://webarchive.nationalarchives.gov.uk/20130107105354/ http:/www.dh.gov.uk/prod_consum_dh/groups/dh_digitalassets/@dh/@ en/documents/digitalasset/dh_4130868.pdf (Accessed 2 December 2017).

DH (DEPARTMENT OF HEALTH). (2012a) Long Term Conditions Compendium of Information. DH 3rd edn. Available at: https://www.gov.uk/government/ news/third-edition-of-long-term-conditions-compendium-published (Accessed 2 December 2017).

DH (DEPARTMENT OF HEALTH). (2012b) *The NHS Mandate. Chapter 2: Enhancing quality of life for people with long-term conditions.* Available at: https://www.gov.uk/government/uploads/system/uploads/attachment_data/ file/256497/13-15_mandate.pdf (Accessed 2 December 2017).

DH (DEPARTMENT OF HEALTH). (2013a) *The NHS Outcomes Framework 2014/15: Domain 2.* Available at: https://www.gov.uk/government/uploads/ system/uploads/attachment_data/file/256456/NHS_outcomes.pdf (Accessed 2 December 2017).

DH (DEPARTMENT OF HEALTH). (2014a) *Transforming primary care: safe, proactive, personalised care for those who need it most.* Available at: https:// www.gov.uk/government/uploads/system/uploads/attachment_data/ file/304139/Transforming_primary_care.pdf (Accessed 2 December 2017)

DH (DEPARTMENT OF HEALTH). (2014b) *Five Year Forward View.* Available at: http://www.england.nhs.uk/wp-content/uploads/2014/10/5yfv-web.pdf (Accessed 2 December 2017).

DH (DEPARTMENT OF HEALTH). (2016) *NHS Outcomes Framework 2016-2017.* Available at: https://www.gov.uk/government/publications/nhs-outcome s-framework-2016-to-2017. (Accessed 2 December 2017).

FRANCIS, J., FISHER, M. and RUTTER, D. (2011) *Reablement: a cost-effective route to better outcomes,* London: Social Care Institute for Excellence. Available at: http://www.scie.org.uk/myscie/almost-there (Accessed 2 December 2017).

GLENDINNING, C., JONE, K., BAXTER, K., RABIEE, P., CURTIS, L., WILDE, A., ARKSEY, H. & FORDER, J. (2010) *Home care re-ablement services: Investigating the longer term impacts.* Working Paper No. DHR 2438.

HM GOVERNMENT. (2010) *Equality Act.* London: HM Government.

IPPR (INSTITUTE FOR PUBLIC POLICY RESEARCH). (2014) *Patients in control: Why people with long-term conditions must be empowered.* Available at: http:// www.ippr.org/assets/media/publications/pdf/patients-in-control_Sept2014.pdf (Accessed 2 December 2017).

LEAHY, R., HOLLAND, S. & McGINN, L. (2012) *Treatment plans and interventions for depression and anxiety disorders.* 2nd edn. London: The Guildford Press.

MANTHORPE, J. (2011) *Benefits of home care reablement in the long term – Community Care.* Community Care. Available at: http://www.communitycare. co.uk/2011/10/06/benefits-of-home-care-reablement-in-the-long-term/ (Accessed 31 August 2014).

NATIONAL INSTITUTE FOR HEALTH AND CARE EXCELLENCE. (2015) *Depression: Summary.* Available at: https://cks.nice.org.uk/depression#!topicsummary (Accessed 2 December 2017).

NAYLOR, C., PARSONAGE, M., MCDAID, D., KNAPP M., FOSSEY, M. & GALEA, A. (2012) *Long term mental health: The cost of co-morbidities.* The Kings Fund Centre for Mental Health. Available at: https://www.kingsfund.org.uk/sites/ default/files/field/field_publication_file/long-term-conditions-mental-health-cost-comorbidities-naylor-feb12.pdf. (Accessed 2 December 2017).

NHS CHOICES. (2015) *Home environment and dementia.* Available at: https:// www.nhs.uk/Conditions/dementia-guide/Pages/dementia-home-environment.aspx (Accessed 2 December 2017).

NHS CHOICES. (2016) *Stress, anxiety and depression: Mindfullness.* Available at: https://www.nhs.uk/Conditions/stress-anxiety-depression/Pages/ mindfulness.aspx (Accessed 2 December 2017).

NHS INFORMATION CENTRE & SOCIAL CARE TEAM (2010) Survey of Carers in Households 2009/10 Gilburt The Health and Social Care Information Centre, Unit Costs of Health and Social Care 2012. Available at: http:// www.ic.nhs.uk/webfiles/publications/009_Social_Care/carersurvey0910/ Survey_of_Carers_in_Households_2009_10_England_NS_Status_v1_0a. pdf/ (Accessed 2 December 2017).

NICE (National Institute for Health and Care Excellence). (2012) *Social care of older people with multiple long-term conditions* – Social Care Guideline. Available at: http://www.nice.org.uk/guidance/gid-scwave0715/ documents/social-care-of-older-people-with-multiple-longterm-conditions-final-scope2 (Accessed 13 September 2013).

RADOMSKI, M. & LATHAM, C. (2008) *Occupational therapy for physical dysfunction.* Philadelphia, PA: Lippincott Williams & Wilkins.

REES, S. (2014) *Physiotherapy works events – coming to you.* The Chartered Society of Physiotherapy. Available at: http://www.csp.org.uk/physioworkslocally (Accessed 3 September 2014).

RIDDAWAY, L. (2012) *Long term conditions strategy and vision.* Northamptonshire NHS Nene clinical commissioning group 2012–2017 version 1.2. Available at: http://www.neneccg.nhs.uk/resources/uploads/files/Long_Term_ Conditions_Strategy_v1_3_17_10__2012%20(1).pdf (Accessed 13 September 2013)

ROSS, S., CURRY, N. & GOODWIN, N. (2011) *Case management: What it is and how it can best be implemented.* London: The King's Fund. Available at: http://www.kingsfund.org.uk/publications/case_management. html (Accessed 13 September 2013)

SAFEGUARDINGUK. (2014) *safeguardinguk.co.uk*. Available at: http://www. safeguardinguk.co.uk (Accessed 31 August 2014).

SCHAFFER, S. K. (2013) *The effect of free personal care for the elderly on informal caregiving. Research pape*r *13/01*, Office of Health Economics. Available at: https://www.ohe.org/publications/effect-free-personal-car e-elderly-informal-caregiving. (Accessed 12 January 2018).

SCIE (SOCIAL CARE INSTITUTE FOR EXCELLENCE). (2012) *At a glance 54: Reablement: a guide for families and carers*. London, United: Author. Available at: http://www.scie.org.uk/publications/ataglance/ataglance54.asp (Accessed 15 January 2018).

SCIE (SOCIAL CARE INSTITUTE FOR EXCELLENCE). (2013a) *Maximising the potential of reablement*. SCIE guide 49. London: Author. Available at: http:// www.scie.org.uk/publications/guides/guide49/ (Accessed 15 January 2018).

SCIE (SOCIAL CARE INSTITUTE FOR EXCELLENCE). (2013b) *Reablement. Module 2: Reablement for care workers*. London: SCIE. Available at: http://www.scie. org.uk/assets/elearning/reablement/module_2_web/index.html (Accessed 10 January 2014).

SKELTON, J. (2013) Why occupational therapists are central to reablement services. *The Guardian*. Available at: http://www.theguardian.com/social -care-network-department-of-health-partner/occupational-therapists -reablement-services (Accessed 31 August 2014).

TEW, J., PLUMMIDGE, G., NICHOLLS, V. & CLARKE, H. (n.d.) *Whole family approaches to reablement in mental health: Scoping current practice*. Birmingham: University of Birmingham.

WANLESS, D. (2006) Social care review: Securing good care for older people taking a long-term view. Available at: http://www.kingsfund.org.uk/ sites/files/kf/field/field_publication_file/securing-good-care-for-older -people-wanless-2006.pdf (Accessed 12 December 2017).

WEBSTER, R. (2014). *Are you ready?* Frontline, p. 21. Available at: http://www. nhsconfed.org (Accessed 10 September 2014).

WHO (WORLD HEALTH ORGANIZATION). (2012). *Health topics: Noncommunicable diseases*. Available at: http://www.who.int/topics/chronic_disease/en/ (Accessed 31 August 2014).

WHO (WORLD HEALTH ORGANIZATION). (2014) *Together we can prevent and control the world's most common diseases*. Available at: http://www. who.int/nmh/publications/ncd-infographic-2014.pdf?ua=1 (Accessed 2 February 2016).

WILDE, A. & GLENDINNING, C. (2012) 'If they're helping me then how can I be independent?' The perceptions and experience of users of home-care re-ablement services. *Health & Social Care in the Community*, vol. 20, no. 6, 583–590.

WINKEL, A., LANGBERG, H. & EJLERSEN, E. (2015) Reablement in a community setting. *Disability and Rehabilitation*, vol. 37, no. 15, 1347–1352.

WONG, P. (2010) Organisational impact of developing reablement services. Master's thesis, University of Chester.

7

Taking Control: The Psychosocial Benefits of Reablement

H. M. Chapman

Chapter overview

This chapter discusses the psychosocial theories that underpin the philosophy and practice of reablement services. Prior to a long-term condition an older person will have fulfilled a role (indeed several) and will have taken an active part in community life (Coulter, Roberts and Dixon 2013). When a person is incapacitated by impairment, disability and pain the natural consequence is that they become a 'user' of health and/or social care services. This change is often dramatic and involves some distress, often associated with the level of importance an individual places on the activities they are no longer able to carry out. In addition, inpatient care can reduce mobility (Merreywether and Chapman 2013), as well as creating dependence on others for personal care and daily activities (see Chapter 4). Alternatively, and with reablement, a person can regain a sense of control over their lives, which includes psychological, social and physical recovery. There is a need for the person to be engaged in a meaningful process which genuinely advances independent living. However, loss of confidence, feelings of helplessness and an altered **self-concept** create barriers to regaining control. Societal expectations of recovery (including those of acute health services) can make long-term illness and disability discreditable experiences, inhibiting social engagement and increasing feelings of helplessness. Together with the person, the attitude of reablement workers (anyone who works with a service user in a reablement capacity) is thus a critical factor in social inclusion (In Control 2015) and reablement.

Concordance, the respectful partnership between service user and service provider in planning and achieving essential aspects of the reablement process, is a fundamental requirement of reablement. It involves valuing the person and acknowledging the human relationship, promoting self-esteem, a sense of control and confidence to try, without worrying about failure. Immanuel Kant, the eighteenth-century philosopher, identified the importance of treating people as ends in themselves, rather than as means to an end (McCormack and McCance 2010), with important implications for the rights of human beings, irrespective of their earning potential, cognitive abilities, appearance, morality or other attributes of difference. Kant also identified the importance of autonomy, and behaving in ways that protected it, in order to promote respect for the self and for other human beings (Gregor 1997). His view of autonomy was that the individual should be free to make a moral choice, rather than come under the influence of more powerful others, and it is from this that the principle of informed consent in modern health and social care is derived (Lysaught 2004). So, in order to respect the service user, we need to support them to make fully informed choices about their reablement plan and then enable them to pursue those choices, even if we would make different ones. Respect for self and others is strongly echoed in the humanistic values of unconditional positive regard, congruence (or authenticity) and empathy, to promote personal growth or self-actualisation. **Unconditional** positive regard means valuing the person as an end in themselves, regardless of their status or personal characteristics. **Congruence** means that a person's view of themselves as they are (self-image) and the way they would like to be (ideal self) are very similar, so the person feels happy with who they are. **Empathy** means understanding the world from the other person's view in order to relate to their emotional feelings and needs. **Self-actualisation**, or personal growth, is the process of leading a life in which the person feels happy within themselves but looks forward to the next challenge or opportunity for self-development. These values are fundamental to the **person-centred** therapy of Carl Rogers (1961) and are used to promote the development of cognitive and emotional adjustment. Thus, the person sees themselves as worthy of respect and is able to plan a future that involves growth and development.

Differing terms are used for the role of the service user in working with health professionals: adherence, compliance and concordance. Compliance suggests unwilling or unthinking obedience, but not taking medicines or following advice, which affects health outcomes and costs, can be a mechanism by which the service user is blamed for any failure to recover (Bissell, May and Noyce 2004), sometimes earning them the label of being 'non-compliant'. Adherence means the active choice to follow the advice or prescription of a health professional, and is the term generally used in relation to pharmacological interventions, while concordance is agreement upon a plan of action or care management which incorporates the knowledge and views of the person and the professional (Horne et al. 2005). Outmoded emphasis on the importance of compliance with health and social care professionals, which creates a barrier to open communication, undermines the value of the individual and reinforces their view of themselves as helpless, leading to dependence and disability. These psycho-emotional dimensions of disability that oppress people are described by Thomas (2004, p. 38) as 'being made to feel of lesser value, worthless, unattractive, or disgusting' and can affect both their self-concept and their understanding of their relationships with others. Consequently, it is essential for all health and social care professionals and support workers who work in reablement to understand these ideas and to value and respect the humanity of the service users with whom they interact.

This chapter will provide an explanation and synthesis of key theoretical concepts that underpin a psychosocial understanding of the issues associated with disability, ageing and long-term conditions. Initially, it will explore the idea of the self, and how the psychology of the self influences human thoughts, feelings and behaviours within, and as a result of, the reablement interaction. This will be followed by a broad discussion of ageing theories such as disengagement, active ageing and **gerotranscendence** as well as elements of positive psychology. Understanding **stigma** will enable understanding of personal values in order to develop non-stigmatising attitudes and behaviour. Centrally, the need to facilitate the personal motivation and **self-efficacy** of service users, while enabling them to feel secure and confident, will illustrate the complexity of working with individuals within the context of reablement.

Chapter objectives

By the end of this chapter you should be able to:

➤ Determine what self-concept is and how it affects the success of reablement and is in turn affected by it

➤ Recognise learned helplessness and how it is reinforced by a loss of control

➤ Outline the ways in which stigma acts as a barrier to reablement

➤ Appraise psychosocial theories of ageing and their implications for reablement

➤ Describe person-centred therapeutic relationships as the foundation of reablement practice

What is our self-concept and where does it come from?

The idea of the self probably seems quite obvious to us as human beings – we are different to other people, but share similar characteristics with them; we see ourselves as existing consistently from one part of our life to another. We may change and develop, but there is a relationship between our childhood self and our adult self. Indeed, older relatives are often keen to remind us of our childhood indiscretions ('You always were impulsive, remember when you...'). So, who are you? List your answers (or draw your self-portrait) in Student Activity Box 7.1:

Student Activity 7.1   Exploring your self-concept

Who am I?

The way you have described yourself (in Student Activity 7.1), or think of yourself, is your **self-concept**. It is your mental representation of yourself, and contains judgements, feelings, attitudes and beliefs about yourself, which affect the way in which you see the world and other people, and so contribute to your personality. You know yourself very well, including the ways in which you think, feel and behave, but sometimes unexpected responses can trigger a re-evaluation of yourself and your value to others.

Where does my self-concept come from?

Our self-concept is the view we have of ourselves as being a certain sort of person with different traits, attributes and characteristics. It develops from our earliest interactions with others, and is dependent on a view of ourselves based on the way others communicate their responses to us. This social self, or view of ourselves as others see us, was first suggested by C. H. Cooley's (1922) idea of the 'looking-glass self', where we imagine what another person thinks or feels about us, and how they will judge us, and include that in our self-concept. So, our assessment of how others see and value us is central to our self-esteem. In Cooley's (1922, pp. 184–185) words, 'we live in the minds of others without knowing it', highlighting how important our views of other people are to them. This socially sensitive self is much less stable than the experiencing self because it is made up of our understanding of how others have seen us in the past. This means that our view of ourselves can alter in response to the way other people react to us, particularly if we value or respect that person. In reablement practice, entering people's homes, we may be seen as 'experts', so our reactions to service users can have a profound influence on their self-concept, particularly where they may have experienced a loss of role in terms of family responsibilities, career or member of a social group. Self-awareness, as well as understanding the feelings of others, is therefore essential for the reablement worker to be effective in promoting biopsychosocial well-being through their encounters.

According to George Herbert Mead's theory of **symbolic interactionism** (Schellenberg 1978), this interaction with others is how we develop a socially sensitive self-as-object or the *'me'*. We learn, through the reactions of others, to react to and assess ourselves in the same way as we do towards other people. To do this, we have to be able to take the role of the other, to internalise it as the 'me'. For example, if we are told that we are a 'good' person every time we tidy up, we will learn to see ourselves as a tidy, and therefore good, person, although a fear of not being seen as good might make us prioritise tidiness over other qualities or activities. Mead proposed that we do this initially through the symbols, gestures, words and sounds that others use towards us. Toddlers talk to themselves aloud in the tone and language that their important others have used to them (for example, 'Tidy up *first*, Jane'). Then, we adopt roles in our pretend play that we may aspire to in adult life, such as parent, teacher, doctor or nurse, and increase our understanding of their motivations. In late childhood and early adolescence, we go through the 'game' stage, where we must take into consideration the views of many different people, the generalised other. In this way, we acquire a variety of social perspectives on ourselves and incorporate them into our sense of self, or self-concept.

Erving Goffman was a sociologist whose work explored the way people's interactions affected, and were affected by, their perceptions of how other people saw them (Goffman 1959). He realised that social status was dependent on how the person presented themselves to others, and by current views in society of what was valued and what was discreditable.

To be discreditable meant that a person lost their good name or reputation, their standing in society, because of something that made them less worthy than others. He introduced the idea that people could be discredited by stigma, either because of a physical illness or disability, even obesity; because of a discreditable trait, such as mental illness, sexual deviancy, alcohol or drug misuse; or because of a tribal identity such as nationality, religion or ethnicity. The effects on the self of being discredited would then lead to them being rejected by others. This would lead to a loss of self-esteem and a loss of value within encounters, meaning that their views would be less believable and less important, and they would be unlikely to achieve the outcomes they wanted. Service users, by definition, need support, and may feel that becoming more dependent, being ill, disabled or older, or in some way different, makes them less creditable. By being aware of these possible feelings, the reablement worker can show, by listening to the person and responding to their lead, that they are valued and respected.

Goffman (1963) also makes the point that people with stigmatising characteristics are socialised, alongside the rest of society, into discrediting people with those characteristics, making it difficult for them not to concur in accepting the stigma as discrediting. If stigma affects the views of service users, it can also affect the views of reablement workers towards them, which is why it is important to be aware of possible stigmas, prejudices and assumptions, in order to overcome them. According to Age UK (Abrams et al. 2011) 64% of people in the UK saw age discrimination as serious, in terms of a lack of respect for people because of their age. This is more important for older people because their self-worth may be negotiated within a small number of interactions where they may be perceived as having lower status, particularly with health and social care workers. Charmaz (1983) argues that one of the factors involved in the loss of self-esteem and self-identity in people with long-term illness is the way they are seen and treated by health professionals. She suggests that, particularly where people are more isolated from society, the interaction with the physician (and by extension other health and social care professionals) assumes greater importance in the co-construction of the self-concept, and concluded that:

> When ill persons receive positive reflections of self in interaction and take them as credible and real, they are more apt to regard themselves positively. But when demeaned and discredited by those to whom they attach significance – even during the briefest of interactions – then maintaining a positive self-image becomes problematic.
>
> (Charmaz 1983, p. 181)

In an unequal situation, people present themselves in a way that they believe is most likely to achieve the outcome that is best for them

(Werner and Malterud 2003), but this can result in embarrassment and loss of self if the health and social care professional does not accept their viewpoint as relevant or valid.

Think about how you feel about yourself, and then think about how going to see a professional about a problem can make you feel (see Student Activity 7.2).

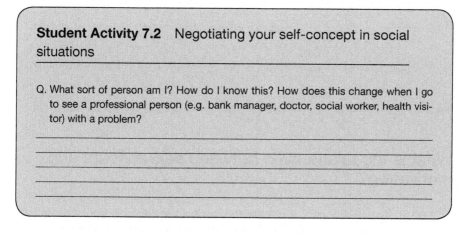

Student Activity 7.2 Negotiating your self-concept in social situations

Q. What sort of person am I? How do I know this? How does this change when I go to see a professional person (e.g. bank manager, doctor, social worker, health visitor) with a problem?

Now, how do service users' self-concepts differ? How might this affect the way they interact with you (personality differences)?

Reflect on your own feelings towards people with different types of illness and disability (Student Activity 7.3) – are there aspects related to appearance, communication skills, temperament, health behaviours or care needs that affect the ways in which you feel and think about a service user?

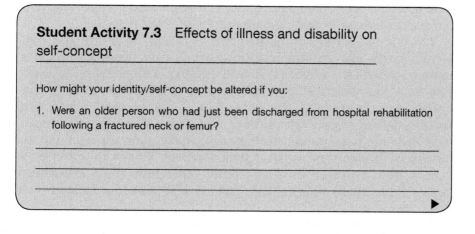

Student Activity 7.3 Effects of illness and disability on self-concept

How might your identity/self-concept be altered if you:

1. Were an older person who had just been discharged from hospital rehabilitation following a fractured neck or femur?

▶

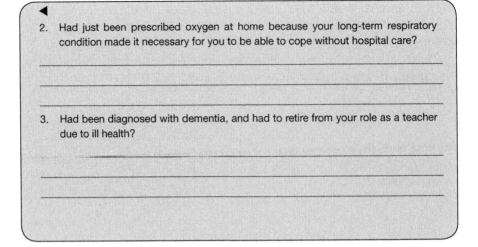

2. Had just been prescribed oxygen at home because your long-term respiratory condition made it necessary for you to be able to cope without hospital care?

3. Had been diagnosed with dementia, and had to retire from your role as a teacher due to ill health?

What is the relationship between self-concept and motivation?

The other part of the self, the experiencing, living-in-the-moment, active self, the 'I', develops from early interactions with the primary caregiver, when babies come to understand that they can affect their environment (including people) because others respond to them *as if* they have intentions and beliefs about their own behaviour (Schaffer 1977). This is when the infant develops a sense of self-efficacy or control over events in the world (Bandura 1997). Just as the child is beginning to realise that objects (including people) still exist even when she can't see them, she also begins to learn that *she* exists separate to others and is a permanent being. At the same time, the infant also starts to see how others react to them, and learns that different behaviours will elicit different responses from others. In adulthood, self-efficacy is strengthened by achievement of our goals, while not achieving goals can make us feel helpless.

Chronic stress has significant negative effects on health and well-being, partly due to the relationship between stress and reduced immunity, which can affect wound healing, vulnerability to infection and even cancer (Kiecolt-Glaser et al. 2002). Thus, stress affects health directly through the physiological effects of the long-term stress response. People who believe they have little personal control over their life have poorer health habits, have more illnesses and are less likely to take steps to treat their illnesses. This is the reverse for people with a greater sense of control. Therefore, stress also affects health indirectly by making them feel helpless to change their lifestyle behaviours in order to improve their health. Conversely, a person's perception that they can cope with perceived environmental stressors prevents the stress response from being activated, while achieving a goal, such as walking for ten minutes, enhances the likelihood of repeating the performance (of walking for ten minutes) another day (Bandura 1997). Once a sense of skill mastery and self-efficacy is gained, the new health behaviours are more likely to be maintained than mere establishment of habit.

Seligman's (1975) theory of learned helplessness

When people suffer from stress over a long period and are unable to escape from it, or if they are unable to achieve the outcomes they want, they begin to feel helpless. Situations of inescapable stress can produce apathy, where people stop striving for goals and come to believe they have no control over their lives, so that even when the opportunity for improvement or escape is offered, they do not take control or move in that direction. Seligman (1975) describes this phenomenon as '**learned helplessness**' – we learn not to try to get what we want because we have learned that we will fail. This is also a key characteristic of depression.

Student Activity 7.4   Reflection on disempowerment and learned helplessness

Think back to school when you had a teacher you didn't like (or who didn't like you), or to a boss for whom everything you did was wrong, or a family member (parent, sibling, partner) who constantly criticised you. How did you feel? What did you do about it eventually, if anything?

However, not everyone who is exposed to uncontrollable negative events develops learned helplessness. Some seem to have greater **resilience**, often using active coping mechanisms to deal with their distress and being mindful of positive aspects of their life. So, while people may be at greater risk of learned helplessness following a serious illness diagnosis or a severe injury, those with self-belief, friendship support and wider social links may feel more able to cope with their situation than those who feel isolated and afraid (Haglund et al. 2007). Depressed people often blame themselves for negative events that are beyond their control and may avoid confronting their difficulties for fear of increasing their feelings of anxiety and low self-esteem. Awareness of the service user's mood, motivation and strengths can aid the reablement worker in being encouraging and setting achievable goals that challenge them without a risk of 'failure'.

A key factor in learned helplessness is that people make different attributions (reach decisions about the causes of events) and judge themselves accordingly. They do this according to three dimensions of the situation (Skinner 1996). First, if the person feels trapped in their helpless situation because they are unable to control it, they are likely to lose self-esteem, but if it is due to something beyond their control, their self-esteem may remain intact, but they are still unlikely to try to overcome the situation. Second, if the negative situation is long-term, such as Type II diabetes, then it is more likely to lead to a sense of helplessness than a short-term problem, such as a broken wrist. Third, they are more likely to feel helpless if they think their situation is caused by a personal attribute, such as 'lack of willpower', rather than something specific to the situation, such as nicotine dependency. For the reablement worker, this underlines the importance of discussing what has caused a goal not to be achieved. It is not caused by a failing in the person, but either by the goal needing refinement or by specific circumstances that can be altered. For example, there may be an intermediate step that needs to be achieved first, or a piece of equipment that would help, or perhaps a rest built into the day so that the service user has more energy for that particular activity when they need to carry it out.

We have known since the 1970s that having control over their lives significantly benefits health, well-being and even lifespan in older people. Seminal research by Rodin and Langer (1977) found that residents in a nursing home who were given plants to care for and were encouraged to make decisions about participating in activities and rearranging furniture lived a happier, more active and longer life than those who were not. Even where people have to give other people control over their money and other life tasks, if they have chosen to do so they feel positive about it, whereas if control is taken from them they have negative outcomes. This means that being in control affects both the ability to perform activities of living and health outcomes, but where support is needed, if it is an agreed, negotiated transfer of control, feelings of helplessness can be avoided (Morgan and Brazda 2013). These principles of choice, negotiated outcomes and control of the process by the service user are fundamental to the practice of reablement.

Psychosocial theories of ageing and stigma

Psychosocial theories focus on the thoughts, feelings and behaviours of the individual and how they are affected by their interactions with others, by their culture and by the systems within society. Ageing can be seen, from a biological perspective, as a decline in a person's appearance and performance. Consequently, ageing may be seen to decrease the value of the person, causing older people to be discredited, ignored and even become victims of abuse. However, such stigma would ignore both individual differences and experiences of each person, and lead to an oversimplification of their reablement needs. It is important to understand psychosocial theories of ageing because:

➢ It is difficult to empathise with elderly patients if we do not have an understanding of their mental perspective.

➢ Often, it is difficult to understand the slowness of body and mind, seeing elderly people as slow, awkward or even a 'burden'. To avoid ageism, we need to understand individual differences and other factors.

➢ What we accept as normal ageing might be caused by unresolved psychological needs which could be met through our assessment and interpersonal/communication skills.

➢ It affects the sort of service which we accept as appropriate for elderly patients.

An early theory of ageing, **disengagement theory** (Cumming, Henry and Damianopoulos 1961), suggests that people gradually withdraw from more powerful roles in society, focusing more on close family or friends, to prevent disruption to society when they die, and to reduce the stress and strain of leading a fuller life. Disengagement is a mutual shift of attention and power from retiring people to the next generation. In this theory, it is seen as normal and functional for older people to lose status in return for a reduction in the demands made on them, and possibly financial or other support from society. However, this model assumes that older people choose to withdraw, rather than feeling less valued within society because they are perceived to have less to offer. Potential consequences of this theory are that it institutionalises ageism within our society, and causes the implicit view that ageing is a discrediting attribute that leads to being stigmatised compared with 'normal' people (Goffman 1963). This increases the likelihood that older people (as with people with long-term conditions) will have lower self-esteem.

An alternative view, the **activity theory of ageing** by Havighurst, Neugarten and Tobin (1968), suggests the maintenance of earlier active patterns of life is associated with successful retirement and that activity helps physical and psychological well-being. While this is a less stigmatising view of ageing, nonetheless, it implies that older people are only valued as long as they are active and do not act as if they are old. For example, in the UK, older people are often referred to as an economic burden, although a recent Northern Ireland (COPNI 2014) report identified that, even taking into account the financial costs of benefits and health care, the monetary and social value (such as childcare) that older people add to the economy is greater than the cost. While this is a welcome alternative view to that of older people being a drain on resources, it still reinforces the view that they are of more value if they contribute economically to society. The activity theory also suggests that older people accept some responsibility for their own ageing, and therefore that those older people who experience physical and psychological ill health may be less deserving of respect than others. This fits in with Graham Scambler's (2006) view that the emphasis on personal responsibility by the UK Government in its welfare policies has resulted in people with long-term conditions and disability being stigmatised and blamed for not overcoming their exclusion from society through self-help strategies. So, the activity theory of ageing can be positive if it challenges our stereotypes of all older people as being physically frail and dependent, but it can lead to discrimination against those older people who have health and social care problems.

Lars Tornstam, who studies the sociology of ageing, found that this view of successful ageing was largely based on a western white middle-class, middle-aged view of success in life, being related to 'activity, productivity, efficiency, individuality, independence, wealth, health, and sociability' (Tornstam 2005, p. 3). However, older people themselves, when asked about their view of successful ageing, are more likely to talk about developing affinity with others across generations and a need for solitude to meditate on things. This idea of gerotranscendence, in which the older person makes choices that suit their needs and desires in later life, may seem similar to disengagement theory, as it appears to suggest a less active role for the older person. However, Tornstam argues that this is not a repackaged disengagement theory, as it is different for each individual, dependent on their own preferences and values, and sees that ageing may allow people to give themselves positive choices to alter their priorities in life. Thus, it is a developmental model of ageing, allowing people to engage with the world on their own terms. This accords with Rogers' theory of lifelong development in order to become the person that one wants to become, and the importance of personal freedom from fear of disapproval in order to achieve this.

The psychology of therapeutic relationships for reablement

In order to promote a feeling of being valued, reduce stress and support the service user to believe that they are able to regain their life skills, the reablement worker needs to establish a trusting relationship with them. Carl Rogers (1961) was interested in helping people with their psychological problems, but he did not agree with a behaviourist viewpoint that if you altered someone's behaviour so that they appeared to be 'normal' then they were. Nor did he agree with the psychoanalytical viewpoint that only the analyst could understand the hidden meanings buried within preconscious thought, such as in dreams, which could unlock the key to someone's personality. Rather, he thought that therapy should be centred on the person finding their own goals and achieving this within a secure professional relationship. We will look at this idea of a secure professional relationship later, but first we need to understand how Rogers (1961) thought people's personalities developed. Rogers (1961) identified that people have two basic needs: self-actualisation and positive regard.

Self-actualisation

Rogers (1961) suggested that everyone needs freedom to grow or become all that they can become. He suggested this was a natural process, which helps people to feel good, and one that could be hindered by negative experiences that made them anxious about trying to change and develop. This self-actualisation is not an endpoint; it is about always having something to aim for – this is what Rogers meant by a good life. How many of you would like to go on a trek in the jungle, achieve a qualification, see your children become successful adults (whatever that is), alter your environment, learn a new skill? By having these goals and trying to achieve them, you are self-actualising. Rogers saw self-actualisation as a basic need that, if thwarted, would *lead* to psychological problems. So, if the service user does not feel that the reablement service is helping them to achieve their goals, then their mental well-being is likely to be affected.

Positive regard

From birth, we all have a basic need for love, respect and approval from other people. Rogers (1961) thought that if we grow up with this positive regard, without having to win it by behaving in a certain way, then we would feel secure in the other person's unconditional love or positive regard. If we feel secure, this frees us to explore the world and our potential to develop within it. However, if we have to behave in certain ways to feel this positive regard (conditional regard), then we grow up to feel that our parents only love this perfectly behaved child that we know is not us, so we do not feel truly loved. Also, we will not risk trying anything new or altering our behaviour, in case we should incur disapproval. For service users who fear that the reablement worker may disapprove of them if they fail in some way, this may lead to them expressing views that they cannot do something and avoiding any activity where weakness might be shown. Clearly, this conditional positive regard can lead to people being so anxious about their self worth that they find it difficult to form relationships with other people. If someone has experienced conditional love in their early development, they are more likely to have conditions of worth – standards which they think are more likely to win approval from others. Since these standards are often very difficult to achieve, they are likely to think that they are unworthy of love or positive regard. In other words, their ideal self and their real self are very different, giving them low self-esteem. The reablement worker could experience this as a service user who does not engage with them or who is more difficult to build a relationship with.

In Rogers' (1961) opinion, this is what often caused the problems that brought people to therapy. He called it **incongruence** between their true inner self and the outer self, which was taking on and acting out a role in order to make the person likeable to others. The low self-esteem and related anxiety this incongruence causes can lead to self-harming behaviours, such as alcohol and drug misuse, hostility towards others, risky behaviours and clinging to any partner or potential partner at the expense of all other needs for self-actualisation. It can also inhibit people from trying to grow and change because of fear of failure in others' view, reflected in their self-esteem. So, some people may be reluctant to engage with reablement in case they 'fail'. However, Rogers (1961) found, through his therapy practice, that developing a trusting relationship allowed the person to achieve congruence, and that this allowed them to overcome long-standing feelings of insecurity and accept themselves, allowing them to grow and self-actualise (become all that they could become). Consequently, the reablement worker has an important role in developing a trusting relationship with the service user, so that they in turn can try new activities and ways of living their life.

This therapeutic relationship is based upon three principles: unconditional positive regard, empathy and authenticity. For **unconditional positive regard**, the professional needs to value and accept the person for who they are, without judging them, enabling them to begin to understand and accept themselves. For **empathy**, the reablement worker needs to see the world of the person from that person's perspective, actively listening to their concerns, checking their own understanding of what the service user means. For **authenticity**, the reablement worker needs to be genuine with the service user, and not 'put on a front' for them, so that it is possible to connect with them as a fellow human being. These conditions for growth enable the person to 'be themselves' and not hide behind Goffman's (1959) mask of playing a role. It takes time for this trust to develop, which is why professional relationships with service users may not be instantly effective and reablement workers need to be resilient in the face of setbacks.

Rogers (1969) applied this person-centred approach to learning, identifying that we can all learn, and are most likely to do so when we see the goal as relevant to us. This is why it is so important for the service user to identify their preferred activity and its meaning for them, as it means they are more likely to achieve their goal. It is also important not to feel that failure would harm us, as we are most creative and independent in our learning when we feel free to experiment. Consequently, the reablement worker needs to be positive about attempting to achieve goals, whether or not they are actually achieved. Rogers (1969) also identified that experiential learning was important, and that when the person wants to learn they will learn and change in a more lasting way. Importantly, he suggested that, once we feel confident in learning in one aspect of our life, we will gain confidence in all learning approaches. This implies that once we support a person to achieve mastery in one area of their life, including making their own choices, they will be more likely to attempt to gain mastery over other aspects of their life. Consequently, an approach that values the person and their autonomy in making choices will enhance their reablement, while any attempt to assume control of the care planning or care intervention will undermine their confidence and lead to feelings of helplessness.

Overview of chapter and application to practice

By asking doctors and patients how much each thinks the doctor respects them, we know that people can accurately assess how respectful health professionals feel towards them (Beach et al. 2006). Patient perceptions of how respected they are affects their trust in the doctor, their adherence to advice and their health outcomes (Martin et al. 2005). Consequently, if reablement workers want service users to work with them to achieve increased satisfaction, well-being, function and autonomy, it is important that they value and respect them. People with a disability, people with long-term conditions (Charmaz 1983) and older people are particularly vulnerable to having their self-esteem affected by the health and social care workers with whom they come into regular contact. Service users identify with cultural values of status and discreditable attributes (Goffman 1963) and are likely to accept negative views of the self, particularly within the dominant western culture that focuses on self-determination, activity and independence (Tornstam 2005; Scambler 2006). Feelings of low self-worth and experiences of feeling devalued can lead to learned helplessness (Seligman 1975) which results in people feeling unable to help themselves and learn new behaviours. The stress they experience as a result from this loss of control also directly affects their health, making them more susceptible to infection, autoimmune disease and cancer, as well as cardiovascular disease such as acute coronary syndrome and stroke. For reablement to be effective, it is necessary for the reablement worker to value and respect the service user in order to promote their self-esteem and motivate them to engage with the process.

People who feel as if they have to behave in a certain way in order to gain approval and be acceptable to others will experience mental distress (Rogers 1961). They will also be inhibited from learning and gaining mastery over new skills (or regaining old ones) (Rogers 1969). The overriding philosophy of reablement is to value every human being equally, irrespective of their needs and abilities. However, individual reablement workers' attitudes develop in accordance with societal values, which influence the value they place on people's personal attributes and abilities. Reablement workers need to overcome these influences on the way they see the service user, and the way the service user sees themselves. By doing so, they will be able to provide person-centred care that allows the service user to feel free to try new ways of achieving their activity goals, often several times before success is achieved. The service user will also feel more in control of the process and therefore more likely to achieve long-lasting beneficial outcomes. People react to feeling undervalued and stressed in different ways: they may withdraw from engagement in an encounter; they may express feelings of hurt, anger and even aggression; they may be acceptant and compliant, resulting in a loss of autonomy. These feelings, and their causes, may be a consequence of previous relationships with others and their sense of security, and may be particular to previous encounters with health and social care professionals. It is important, therefore, not to react defensively or judgementally when you perceive a service user to be reacting unfairly towards you. This will create a barrier that will prevent you from empathising with the person, seeing their point of view and being able to develop a trusting relationship with them. That trusting relationship is necessary for you to develop a concordant approach to their reablement, in which you share common goals and work as partners to achieve them. Therefore, it is important to actively listen to the service user and engage with them as a person in order to demonstrate that they are valued and central to the reablement encounter. This empathy is one of the three requirements for a person-centred encounter.

Engaging with people in a valuing way can only be achieved by the reablement worker if they are congruent, that is, they know themselves well and are reasonably happy with the person they are, so they are able to be genuine with the service user, rather than hiding behind a professional role. This does not mean sharing personal details or becoming informal friends with a service user, it just means not putting on a false front. As we know, service users know when they are valued, so congruence makes a reablement worker more trustworthy, and therefore is likely to lead to a more trusting relationship. However, since being known to oneself and liking oneself is essential for congruence, this means that reablement workers need to develop skills of self-awareness through reflection and (clinical) supervision.

Therapeutic relationships are also built on unconditional positive regard, which cannot be achieved if reablement workers hold contradictory attitudes of stigma and value certain types of people less than others. Therefore, it is important to analyse our own values and attitudes towards people, to see if we are influenced by views that we have heard expressed in the media, or by politicians or other powerful people, and evaluate whether they accord with our core philosophy of valuing all people equally and non-judgementally. Stigma is a constant within society, with people seeking to increase their own value to society, and therefore their own status in it, by identifying attributes that they do not hold, or individuals whom they perceive as different to them, as discredited. Once this stigma is accepted, a whole group of people becomes devalued and discriminated against within society. Both reablement workers and service users are influenced by stigma, so it is important not only to raise awareness of stigma in ourselves and others, but to actively challenge it in ourselves and others. By valuing our service users, we underline our own value to society in reabling people to self-actualise and become all that they can become.

Summary

➤ Autonomy is essential for personal growth and mental well-being, and is fundamental to effective reablement.

➤ Autonomy can only be promoted effectively if the service user feels valued by the reablement worker.

▶

◀

➤ Feelings of low self-esteem inhibit service user confidence and development, leading to learned helplessness and further health problems.

➤ Attitudes towards certain attributes can lead to stigmatising of people who are old, disabled or otherwise different. These attitudes are culturally learned, and reablement workers may not be aware of their own stigmatising attitudes.

➤ For support workers to value others, they must develop self-awareness and self-esteem through reflection and clinical supervision.

➤ Active listening and empathy are essential attributes in promoting self-esteem.

➤ Valuing others has the potential to enhance self-worth.

Recommended reading

HEFFERON, K. & BONIWELL, I. (2011) *Positive psychology: Theory, research and applications.* Maidenhead: Open University Press.

References

ABRAMS, D., RUSSELL, P. S., VAUCLAIR, C.-M. & SWIFT, H. (2011) *A snapshot of ageism in the UK and across Europe.* European Research Group on Attitudes to Age, University of Kent. London: Age UK.

BANDURA, A. (1997) Self-efficacy and health behaviour. In A. Baum, S. Newman, J. Weinman, R. West & C. McManus (eds) *Cambridge handbook of psychology, health and medicine.* Cambridge: Cambridge University Press.

BEACH, M. C., ROTER, D. L., WANG, N.-Y., DUGGAN, P. S., & COOPER, L. A. (2006) Are physicians' attitudes of respect accurately perceived by patients and associated with more positive communication behaviors? *Patient Education and Counseling*, vol. 62, no. 3, 347–354.

BISSELL, P., MAY, C. R. & NOYCE, P. R. (2004) From compliance to concordance: barriers to accomplishing a re-framed model of health care interactions. *Social Science & Medicine*, vol. 58, no. 4, 851–862.

CHARMAZ, K. (1983) Loss of self: A fundamental form of suffering in the chronically ill. *Sociology of Health & Illness*, vol. 5, no. 2, 168–195.

COOLEY, C. (1922) *Human nature and the social order (Revised edition).* New York: Scribners. Available at: https://brocku.ca/MeadProject/Cooley/Cooley_1902/Cooley_1902toc.html (Accessed 5 December 2017).

COPNI (COMMISSIONER FOR OLDER PEOPLE IN NORTHERN IRELAND). (2014) *Appreciating age: Valuing the positive contributions made by older people in Northern Ireland.* Belfast: COPNI.

COULTER, A., ROBERTS, S. & DIXON, A. (2013) *Delivering better services for people with long-term conditions: Building the house of care.* London: The King's Fund. Available at: https://www.kingsfund.org.uk/sites/default/files/field/field_publication_file/delivering-better-services-for-people-with-long-term-conditions.pdf (Accessed 4 February 2018).

CUMMING, E., HENRY, W. E. & DAMIANOPOULOS, E. (1961) A formal statement of disengagement theory. In E. Cumming & W. E. Henry (eds) *Growing old: The process of disengagement.* New York: Basic Books, pp. 210–218.

GOFFMAN, E. (1959) *The presentation of self in everyday life.* New York: Doubleday.

GOFFMAN, E. (1963) *Stigma: Notes on the management of spoiled identity.* Englewood Cliffs, NJ: Prentice-Hall.

GREGOR, M. (ed.). (1997) *Kant: Groundwork of the methaphysics of morals.* Cambridge: Cambridge University Press.

HAGLUND, M. E. M., NESTADT, P. S., COOPER, N. S., SOUTHWICK, S. M. & CHARNEY, D. S. (2007) Psychobiological mechanisms of resilience: Relevance to prevention and treatment of stress-related psychopathology. *Development and Psychopathology*, vol. 19, no. 3, 889–920.

HAVIGHURST, R. J., NEUGARTEN, B. L., & TOBIN, S. S. (1968) Disengagement and patterns of aging. In B. L. Neugarten (ed.), *Middle age and aging: A reader in social psychology.* Chicago: University of Chicago Press, pp. 161–172.

HORNE, R., WEINMAN, J., BARBER, N., ELLIOTT, R., MORGAN, M., CRIBB, A. & KELLAR, I. (2005) *Concordance, adherence and compliance in medicine taking.* London: National Coordinating Centre for the Service Delivery and Organisation (NCCSDO). Available at: https://www.researchgate.net/profile/Ian_Kellar/publication/271443859_Concordance_Adherence_and_Compliance_in_Medicine_Taking/links/54cfdb790cf298d65665b4d4.pdf (Accessed 4 February 2018).

IN CONTROL (2018) Our Ethical Values. Available at: http://www.in-control.org.uk/about-us/our-ethical-values.aspx (Accessed 4 February 2018).

KIECOLT-GLASER, J. K., MCGUIRE, L., ROBLES, T. F. & GLASER, R. (2002) Emotions, morbidity, and mortality: New perspectives from psychoneuroimmunology. *Annual Review of Psychology*, vol. 53, no. 1, 83–107.

LYSAUGHT, M. T. (2004) Respect: Or, how respect for persons became respect for autonomy. *Journal of Medicine and Philosophy*, vol. 29, no. 6, 665–680.

MCCORMACK, B. & MCCANCE, T. (2010) *Person-centred nursing: Theory and practice.* Chichester: Wiley-Blackwell.

MARTIN, L. R., WILLIAMS, S. L., HASKARD, K. B. & DIMATTEO, M. R. (2005) The challenge of patient adherence. *Therapeutics and Clinical Risk Management*, vol. 1, no. 3, 189–199.

MERREYWETHER, J. & CHAPMAN, H.M. (2013) Attitudes of nursing staff to inpatient mobilisation: A literature review. *New Scholar: The Journal for Undergraduates of Health and Social Care*, vol. 1, no. 1, 24–28.

MORGAN, L. A. & BRAZDA, M. A. (2013) Transferring Control to Others: Process and Meaning for Older Adults in Assisted Living. *Journal of Applied Gerontology*, vol. 32, no. 6, 651–668.

RODIN, J. & LANGER, E. J. (1977) Long-term effects of a control-relevant intervention with the institutionalized aged. *Journal of Personality and Social Psychology*, vol. 35, no. 12, 897–902.

ROGERS, C. R. (1961) *On becoming a person: A therapist's view of psychotherapy.* Boston, MA: Houghton Mifflin.

ROGERS, C. R. (1969) *Freedom to learn: A view of what education might become.* Columbus, OH: Charles E. Merrill.

SCAMBLER, G. (2006) Sociology, social structure and health-related stigma. *Psychology, Health & Medicine,* vol. 11, no. 3, 288–295.

SCHAFFER, H. R. (1977) *Studies in mother–infant interaction: Proceedings of the Loch Lomond Symposium, Ross Priory, University of Strathclyde, September, 1975.* London: Academic Press.

SCHELLENBERG, J. A. (1978) *Masters of social psychology: Freud, Mead, Lewin, and Skinner.* New York: Oxford University Press.

SELIGMAN, M. E. P. (1975) *Helplessness: On depression, development, and death.* San Francisco, CA: W.H. Freeman.

SKINNER, E. A. (1996) A guide to constructs of control. *Journal of Personality and Social Psychology*, vol. 71, no. 3, 549–570.

THOMAS, C. J. (2004) Developing the social relational in the social model of disability: A theoretical agenda, In C. Barnes & G. Mercer (eds) *Implementing the social model of disability: Theory and research.* Leeds: The Disability Press, pp. 32–47.

TORNSTAM, L. (2005) *Gerontranscendence: A developmental theory of positive aging.* New York: Springer.

WERNER, A. & MALTERUD, K. (2003) It is hard work behaving as a credible patient: Encounters between women with chronic pain and their doctors. *Social Science & Medicine,* vol. 57, no. 8, 1409–1419.

8

Technological Advances in Reablement

G. Ward, E. Rose and S. Whitley

Chapter outline

This chapter will discuss the important role that technology has within the context of reablement in facilitating people to live as independently as possible within their own home. As identified in earlier chapters the demand for support of those with long-term health conditions is set to grow rapidly over the next 15 years and beyond. If the National Health Service (NHS) and social care organisations are to continue to offer high standards of health and care services, they will need to make better and more integrated use of technology to meet the increasing demand for home-based care. Technological advances continue to develop rapidly within western societies and therefore new ways of working need to be considered, while at the same time recognising the requirement for new skills and knowledge in the workforce.

A survey by the Association of Directors of Adult Social Services in England (2013) showed that directors of adult social services had to plan to save another £800 million in the months leading up to April 2014 (145 out of 152 top-tier social services authorities responded). Two of the most marked **trends** indicated by the survey show that 13% of the planned savings (£104 million) will result in direct withdrawal of services, while nearly a fifth of councils thought that a reduction in the levels of personal budgets would be 'highly important'. Given the resource and budget restrictions that are affecting health and social care provision, it is likely that the emphasis on the utilisation of technology will grow as an affordable and acceptable way of supporting people at home. While this is seen as a potentially viable solution, it is not without some contention.

Chapter objectives

➤ Review the potential of technology within reablement

➤ Examine the evidence base for the use of technology

➤ Consider the need for the use of mainstream technology as a means of support and empowerment as service users age in place

➤ Provide examples of how specialist technologies might be used within the context of reablement

➤ Consider the acceptability of technology and the significance of matching the person's need with an appropriate technological solution and the importance of this in reducing abandonment of the technology

➤ Highlight the need for training of health and social care professionals and the integration of technology into practice, including risk management

➤ Review the future of smart home technology within reablement

Defining assistive technology and opportunities within reablement

Awang and Ward (2011) reviewed the emerging definitions of **assistive technology** over a ten-year period, with a preference for that adopted by the Royal Commission on Long-Term Care (1999, p. 325):

> An umbrella term for any device or system that allows an individual to perform a task they would otherwise be unable to do or increases the ease and safety with which the task can be performed.

This definition emphasises inclusivity and the benefits to the wider population with the focus on the enabling nature of assistive technology, rather than it being designed for a particular group of people or disability. It also supports the underpinning philosophy of reablement as being: 'the achievement of goals set by the user and reablement team together, with the overall aim of maximising the user's independence, choice and quality of life, and reducing their need for support in future' (OPM and NEIEP 2010, p. 4). The valuable role that technology can play alongside reablement was further outlined by the Rt. Hon Andrew Lansley MP,

Secretary of State for Health, in his speech on 'The Principles of Social Care Reform', in July 2010:

> We must place renewed emphasis on keeping people as independent as possible, for as long as they feel able, not least by providing earlier support. People need to feel help is there as soon as problems occur ... We have to maximise the potential of **reablement, telecare** and other innovations which can dramatically improve people's lives while also being highly efficient. Some local authorities have picked up this challenge, others have not. We need to accelerate this change so that these services and this approach is the norm.
>
> (The National Archives 2010, emphasis added)

Understanding the development and awareness of the use of technology, within both public and professional arenas, has been hampered by a plethora of terms and definitions to describe these emerging products and services. Doughty and colleagues (2007) reviewed how terminology has developed within assistive technology and proposed three major categories to help define developments – assistive technology, telecare and telehealth.

Assistive technology – refers to fixed or portable adaptations or community equipment that may be mechanical or not and may have electronic components (Doughty et al. 2007). Examples of devices include those to help people with mobility and perform tasks such as cooking, dressing and grooming, such as kitchen implements with large, cushioned grips to help people with weakness or arthritis in their hands; medication dispensers with alarms to help people remember to take their medicine on time, or memory prompting devices that remind someone when an appointment is due.

Telecare – involves use of personal alarms and environmental sensors to enable people to remain safe and independent in their own home for longer. Previously known as community alarms, these systems have developed in both their sophistication and use of new technologies and are now generally referred to as telecare. Telecare offers a wide range of options ranging from simple pendants, which trigger a pager worn by a carer in another part of the home, to environmental sensors, such as motion, fall, fire and gas detectors which dial, via a telephone line, directly to a 24-hour monitoring centre that provides an appropriate response. However, telecare should be as much about the philosophy of dignity and independence as it is about equipment and services (DH 2005).

Sensor technology has also been extended to activity or lifestyle monitoring systems as described by Awang and Ward (2011). These systems typically make use of passive infrared (PIR) movement detectors and other environmental sensors that are triggered as a person moves around their home. Data from the sensors are sent to a web server. Family members or professionals can log on to a password-protected website to view daily activity patterns. An example of this is called the 'Just Checking' system and is discussed in more depth in the section titled 'Specialist technologies'.

Other types of technology such as environmental control systems (ECS) help people with severe disabilities maintain or increase their independence within their own home by offering the means to operate electrical, home security and domestic appliances (Medical Devices Agency 1995). Augmentative and alternative communication (AAC) devices to assist individuals that have limited or absent verbal or non-verbal abilities clearly have a role within reablement and will require the health or social care practitioner to have knowledge of local referral pathways to access these services for specialist assessment. However technological developments, remote control of environments and home automation alongside accessible communication aids within PCs and tablets are bringing cheaper and more accessible alternatives to people (see the section on 'Mainstream technology').

Telehealth – The Royal College of Nursing (2013) defines telehealth as:

> the remote monitoring of physiological data e.g. temperature and blood pressure that can be used by health professionals for diagnosis or disease management. Examples of telehealth devices include blood pressure monitors, pulse oximeters, spirometers, weighing scales and blood glucometers.

The term telemedicine is also used to describe the use of communication and information technologies to deliver clinical care where the individuals involved are not at the same location (Cochrane Library 2010), for example providing advice by telephone, using videoconferencing to discuss a diagnosis, or capturing and sending images for diagnosis. However, this type of communication is equally appropriate for use within reablement services where practitioners may provide support and coaching to service users to encourage behaviour change, via Skype for example. This may be particularly useful in rural areas where poor local transport and transport costs can lead to missed appointments and difficulties in accessing services.

Evidence for the use of technology

The absence of good-quality research and information about cost and clinical effectiveness has been a major reason why telecare has not become embedded as a routine service across the UK (Awang and Ward 2011), although small-scale studies have indicated that telecare and telehealth technology could provide a number of benefits for service users and those with long-term conditions. For example, in Scotland the National Telecare Development Programme (TDP) estimated savings to be over £11 million. In the evaluation report it was estimated that over 81,000 bed days were saved in Scotland in only one year as a result of the telecare services that were installed (York Health Economics Consortium and The Scottish Government 2009).

The Whole System Demonstrator (WSD) programme was set up by the Department of Health in 2008 to provide a clear evidence base to support investment and to show how technology could support people to live independently, and take control and responsibility for their own health and care. The WSD programme is the largest randomised control trial of telehealth and telecare in the world, involving 6,191 patients and 238 GP practices across three sites: Newham, Kent and Cornwall (DH 2011, pp. 1–2). The initial headline findings indicated that, if used correctly, telehealth could deliver a 15% reduction in A&E visits, a 20% reduction in emergency admissions, a 14% reduction in elective admissions, a 14% reduction in bed days and an 8% reduction in tariff costs and also demonstrated a 45% reduction in mortality rates (DH 2011, p. 3). The subsequent research paper (Steventon et al. 2012) concluded that telehealth was associated with lower mortality and emergency admission rates. The analysis, however, of the telecare part of the trial – to assess the impact of telecare on the use of social and health care (Steventon et al. 2013) – found that telecare, as implemented in the WSD trial, did not lead to significant reductions in service use over 12 months. In addition, there was no difference between the intervention and control groups in terms of hospital admissions, although this is only one theme within the analysis, and other evaluation themes will assess effects on quality of life and the views of service users and carers. A cost-effectiveness study will estimate the cost of the telecare intervention (not included so far) and capture services such as community nursing, social work and paramedics. As this is the first large randomised study of the effectiveness of telecare the findings have implications for resource use and planning but the authors recommend that service decisions should also reflect findings from other themes from the evaluation, such as those relating to quality of life.

Mainstream technology

The term mainstream technology refers to any technology that is intended for general use rather than for use by people with disabilities. Mainstream technologies include personal computers, mobile phones, tablets, kitchen gadgets and appliances, for example. All of these have a role within the context of reablement. Applications include the use of memory prompts, GPS location devices and voice-activated controls. According to Jana (2009) mainstreaming has a long history and she cites how Thomas Edison saw his invention of the phonograph as a means of accessing books for people with sight loss by recording book readings. Jana (2009) goes on to highlight how the algorithms that finish words people type in search engines, or e-mail within predictive-text software, have their beginnings in technology. The original aim of algorithms was to support people with disabilities to access computer software. Apple products are widely recognised for being devices that are easy to use and well designed. Some features such as the iPhone's or iPad's voice control evolved from software Apple created to help disabled people use computers in the late 1980s. This was when the developer decided to try to embed 'universal access' in its Macintosh PC line (Jana 2009).

Smartphones and their applications are capable of providing useful support to a range of vulnerable groups, including people with sensory disabilities, those with long-term conditions, such as diabetes or epilepsy, and people with mental health problems or communication difficulties. It is likely that mobile care services using smartphones will be offered in tandem with home telecare services to extend the independence of the service user from the home to the outside environment (Doughty 2011). In-built mobile phone technology facilitates low-cost, downloadable applications that enable the camera, the microphone, the accelerometer, the GPS receiver and the touchscreen within a mobile phone to be used for specific assistive purposes.

The health industry is responding to the increasing popularity and availability of tablets and smartphones, with health and well-being applications estimated to make up approximately 40% of new smartphone apps currently being developed (Smallman 2012). This is a substantial market and only set to increase as the benefits become more apparent and smartphone and tablet technology becomes even more widespread. Health and well-being apps have the potential to be used by health and social care professionals and users, helping to revolutionise the sector and reflect the digital age we live in.

Yet so far telecare and telehealth have yet to be accepted as mainstream services to support people in their own homes. Lack of awareness and confusion over the language and terminology used are hampering the uptake of services. A report by Carers UK found that when the public were asked whether they would use telecare – without giving a definition of what it was – only one in eight (12%) of all respondents said they would use telecare, dropping to only 7% for over 65s. Yet when provided with a definition in plain English, 79% said they would use telecare (Carers UK 2013).

Government initiatives such as the Dallas project (delivering assisted living lifestyles at scale), launched by the Assisted Living Innovation Platform, aimed to act as a large-scale demonstrator of independent living products and services (Technology Strategy Board 2011). This was to show how assisted living technologies and services could promote well-being and help people to live independently across communities throughout the UK. Their target was to positively impact on the lives of 169,000 people by June 2015. The programme was jointly funded by the National Institute for Health Research and the Scottish Government, and the Dallas programme aimed to encourage and help businesses take advantage of this opportunity by engaging them in new service developments with health and social care. The website with updates can be accessed at: https://connect.innovateuk.org/web/dallas.

There is also a growing emphasis on the use of direct payments, personal budgets and a consumer market to enable people to purchase an increasingly affordable and available range of assistive technology, much of which is being produced for consumer consumption (Awang and Ward 2011). However, health and social care professionals will need to have a good awareness of the products and services available in order to be able to signpost service users and carers appropriately and be familiar and comfortable with the use of the technology themselves.

Specialist technologies

Since the 1990s, around the time of the NHS Community Care Act (Legislation.Gov.UK, reprint 2000) there has been a significant government push towards keeping people independent in their own homes. The White Paper 'Our Health, Our Care, Our Say' (DH 2006) documents the vision to move health and social care closer to a person's home rather than hospitals or clinics. Technology can support this through the implementation of telecare and telehealth among other specialist systems.

The development of new integrated technologies is offering exciting and innovative opportunities within reablement. One area currently under development is that of the smart kitchen. This concept has resulted from the acknowledgement that providing care 24/7 can be exhausting (Lindsay 2013). Many hours are spent supporting people to prepare meals but the introduction of smart kitchens aims to reduce the amount of time spent on care and increase the time available for quality contact through promotion of independence. An *Ambient Kitchen* was motivated by the clinical problem of prompting people in the early stages of dementia through multistep tasks (Wherton and Monk 2008). The kitchen environment integrates data projectors, cameras, radio frequency identification tags and readers, object-mounted accelerometers and under-floor pressure sensing using a combination of wired and wireless networks (Oliver et al. n.d.). The aim is that the kitchen is able to detect the activities which occur within it and provide relevant prompts and guidance. For example, it can detect which utensils are being used and how, via embedded accelerometers, which page a recipe book is opened to and project relevant information and instructions onto the wall. It is hoped that this concept will expand to be able to identify potential recipes based upon the ingredients that have been recognised as being selected and put onto the worktop. This would assist those with poor memory, sequencing or planning skills to be able to create a meal or snack independently and therefore has a clear application within reablement.

Smart fridges are becoming more widely available. They have touch-screens or barcode scanners which generate an inventory of the contents and will automatically add items to the user's online shopping account when stocks run low, so assisting people with reduced memory to purchase all their necessities. These fridges are even able to make suggestions for recipes based on the contents.

The Voluntary Organisations Disability Group (2013) argues that the role of AT should be seen to complement a range of interventions to support both families and individuals. All too often family members report that their role has changed from that of a parent, sibling or child to that of a carer, which can have a significant impact upon family dynamics. As many authorities only offered services to those who had critical or substantial care needs (Fair Access to Care) (SCIE 2013) prior to 2014, it often fell to friends and family to complete 'check calls' thus reducing the amount of quality time spent with the family. At the advent of the Care Act 2014 (DH 2014) there was more emphasis on protecting carers' needs (see Chapter 3, 'Model two: Intake and assessment reablement service'). Technological advances in monitoring systems have reduced the need for these check calls, providing 'round the clock reassurance' (Burke 2010), so enabling the family to resume their roles.

These systems operate through the use of PIR sensors which are located around a property. Patterns of behaviour can be monitored, thus indicating whether a person is out of bed or has accessed the kitchen and so on. An example of this technology is the above-mentioned 'Just Checking' which provides information about patterns of daily activity that can indicate a loved one is getting on with their daily life without losing their privacy or having intrusive 'check' visits.

Scenario 8.1   Early stage dementia: Mrs Thomas

Mrs Thomas has early stage dementia. Her family are concerned about her increased level of fatigue during the day. A monitoring system was put in place, as it had been highlighted that Mrs Thomas was getting out of bed in the middle of the night to use the bathroom and then not returning. Once this pattern of behaviour was established appropriate actions were taken to alter her medication and care package to support her into a healthier daily routine, so enabling her to function throughout the day.

Scenario 8.2   A person-centred assistive device: Mr Peters

Mr Peters is 74 years old and has a history of falls. He is a determined man who likes his independence. He refuses to wear a fall detector. He became frustrated with the number of times his family would call to check on his well-being. This was affecting his relationship with his daughter. Since the installation of an activity monitoring system Mr Peters has been able to continue with his day-to-day life without the need for frequent visits. This is because his daughter is able to see that he is active around his property.

Unlike many other systems, this does not raise an alarm if unusual patterns occur. It relies on specified people to log in and review the activity chart (see Figure 8.1). As well as having peace of mind, being able to monitor a loved one remotely provides both the individual and his/her family with greater independence. Jarrold and Yeandle (2009) reiterate the positive effect that such technology can have on carers. They report that carers are more relaxed and confident when systems are in place. It allows the carer to have a break and in some cases even return to paid employment.

As part of an assessment process health and social care professionals should consider the impact that technology could have on someone's life. For the individual, technology such as pendant alarms, fall detectors and epilepsy sensors can boost confidence as they know that they can summon help when needed. Bogus caller alarms, key safes and tracking devices can promote security, and individuals can gain control over their environment through systems that allow them to switch on the television or radio and open windows and so forth without support. Telehealth technology means that a person does not have to make numerous trips to the GP practice to have their blood pressure or glucose levels checked – it can all be done from the home.

Bedroom:

went to bed,
got up and whether
they had a
disturbed night...

Kitchen:

visited the kitchen
to prepare meals...

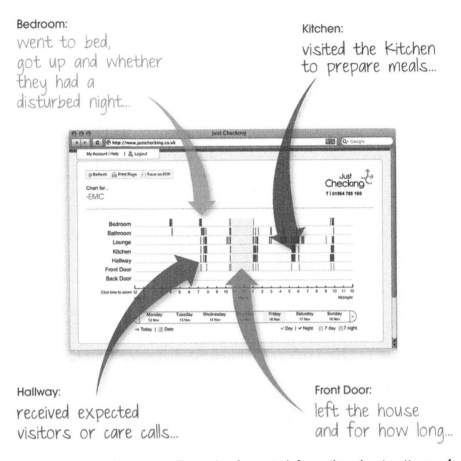

Hallway:

received expected
visitors or care calls...

Front Door:

left the house
and for how long...

Figure 8.1 Just Checking – Example of remote information about patterns of daily activity
Source: From Justchecking.com (accessed 15 January 2014)

However, there are ethical implications to consider when recommending AT. We need to consider the impact that technology can have on an individual, and whether he or she has the capacity to consent to such intervention. The Social Care Institute for Excellence (SCIE 2013) recognises the benefits of AT but also highlights the potential it has to threaten a user's privacy. This is why gaining informed consent is so important.

The potentially isolating effect AT can have is also raised by SCIE (2013), with loneliness being a common theme throughout the chapters in this book. On occasions the carer is the only person that an individual physically sees throughout the day so the impact of replacing this contact with the installation of technology needs to be considered carefully. It is highlighted that AT should not be considered as an alternative to direct social contact unless requested by the client; however, social care services should not be considered purely as a social interaction, and other opportunities to meet this need should be explored.

Acceptance of technology

Consent for the use of AT is no different from the consent required for any other form of intervention. As a health or social care professional you must always ensure that your client has agreed to the installation of equipment and understood its purpose. As practitioners, we may feel that AT is the best solution for our client, but in order for it to work and reduce the level of abandonment, the person needs to accept it.

The Technology Acceptance Model, first developed by Davis in 1989, highlights how a person's perceived usefulness of the product and the perceived ease of use, along with their attitude and intention to use it, greatly impact upon the actual use of a system. So, if someone perceives technology as complicated, they may not wish to engage; if they do not see that the product would be useful, they will not want it. This could have an impact upon the reablement approach, as a person may continue to be dependent upon others as a result of declining technological support.

Culture may also impact upon acceptance; for example, a study of the Asian community in north-west Kent (Milne and Seabrooke 2004) shows how few Asian families utilise support services for relatives with dementia. Clearly this is only a small sample, but it demonstrates that some cultures may not readily accept AT services as they would rather provide the care themselves.

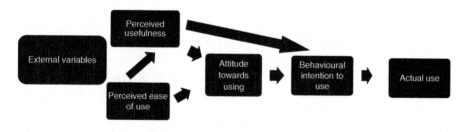

Figure 8.2 Technology Acceptance Model

Source: Davis (1989)

Age may also influence whether technology is accepted. If we consider a person with poor memory, some people from younger generations may be willing to use smartphones and apps to support them and use mobile phone calendar functions to send reminders to their phone, whereas older people may prefer to use a calendar that hangs on the kitchen wall. However, as the generations progress the use of technology is becoming more prevalent. For example, Generation X is the term given to those born between 1965 and 1980. As the first generation to grow up with computers, technology has become part of their lives. As we move through into Generation Y (those born from the mid-1980s), the use of technology is expanding further still. This group of people grew up with technology around them and rely on it to perform many aspects of their lives from work through to social contact. Smartphone permeation has risen to 62% of the population and these smartphone owners are becoming increasingly reliant on their devices, with 54% searching on their smartphones every day (IPSOS MediaCT 2013).

According to the IPSOS survey of 1,000 users of the internet in the UK, adults aged 35–64 account for 53% of smartphone users. This means that those who are most likely to be caring for or supporting older relatives or approaching older age themselves are already familiar with these devices and will expect or demand that information is available via this media to allow them to make decisions and choices about health and well-being.

Reflection Point 8.1   Being without daily access to computers, smartphones and tablets

Think about your own use of computers, tablets and smartphones; imagine the inconvenience and frustration if none of these were available to you and consider the contribution they make to the way you live your life.

Age UK (n.d.) completed a Technology and Older Peoples Evidence Review. It states that the number of people aged 65 and above with access to the internet is rapidly increasing, and those who have access use it more frequently than any other age group to find information and advice, support and services as well as for social interaction. The most recent Office for National Statistics Report (cited in Age UK n.d.) states that 52% of people aged 55–64 in the UK purchased goods over the internet in the last year compared to 22 per cent of people aged 65 and over. The rise since 2008 is higher in these older age groups than the average. This empowers older people to take control of their lives in areas which previously could have been lost; for example, embracing the technology could enable a person to continue shopping even when he or she cannot access the shops independently, as this could be completed online, so maintaining control and independence. It is also noted that 20% of people aged 65 and over downloaded films and music from the internet, rather than ordering them by post. Fifteen per cent of people aged 65 and over did so for e-books, newspapers, magazines and learning materials.

This shift in the uptake of technology will have a significant impact on the opportunities available within a reablement approach and the potential solutions for individuals. As practitioners, we need to be aware of the tech-savvy culture that is developing and ensure that we are abreast of developments and offer appropriate solutions.

Social influences are acknowledged by Venkatesh and colleagues (2003) in their unified theory of acceptance and use of technology. An example of this from experience is when a teenager refused to use a cumbersome communication aid which would have been fixed to her wheelchair for all to see. Instead she opted for a communication app where she could type a text message which would be read out for her, meaning that no special equipment was required, just a phone, just like her peers of a similar age. This demonstrates how reablement needs to be approached on an individual basis, exploring solutions that are acceptable and successful for each person. It may not always be through specialist equipment. As practitioners, we need to think outside the box and utilise everyday items and technology in innovative ways to enable our service users to lead independent lives.

Due to the rapid development of technology, consumers often report that they feel overwhelmed and confused when having to make decisions from a wide range of options, functions and features (MPT 2013). As health and social care professionals we can help to alleviate this confusion through the administration of accurate assessments, ensuring that the person and the technology are compatible. One such assessment tool is the Matching Person and Technology process (MPT 2013). This process takes into consideration the environment in which the technology will be used, as well as the individual's abilities and preferences. The instruments developed within the MPT process are goal-driven so encouraging the practitioner and client to work in partnership, a key element of the reablement approach. Quality of life remains the core focus while practitioners are guided to consider possible solutions. Any mismatches between proposed AT and the potential user are identified in time to reduce the likelihood of abandonment and frustration. The most appropriate solution is established and relevant training given in order for the individual to fully understand the technology, again reducing the possibility of abandonment. It is important to remember that each service user is different and views on technology will vary, so although as practitioners we may have seen a particular piece of equipment prove successful with one person, it does not mean it will be successful with another. In order to be person-centred and promote the service user's engagement in the reablement process we must remain open-minded and solution-focused, working in collaboration with the person to achieve the best possible outcomes.

Student Activity 8.1   Older people and technology

Think about an older person you know – possibly a relative such as a grandparent – who does not use a computer, or have a mobile phone. What might be some of the ways you could talk with them about how their independence could be enhanced by learning to use such devices?

Training of health and social care professionals, integration of technology and practice

It is clear that health and social care services have changed as a result of the rapid and ongoing development of assistive and information technologies (IT) (Carneiro 2006; HSJ 2012). The use of telecare, telehealth and telecommunications technology is facilitating the national agenda in shifting the focus of health care from the hospital setting into the community, allowing a wider range of health and care services to be supported.

Ongoing advances in IT have been key to implementing telehealth technologies which, according to Goodwin (2010), have the potential to improve quality of life, reduce unnecessary hospital and care home admissions, and support care integration by providing care and disease management from multidisciplinary care teams that are linked remotely to patients.

Current problems plaguing contemporary health and social care services, including access, quality, resource distribution and cost containment, have contributed to assistive technology's economic, social and political appeal (Chau and Hu 2002; Carneiro 2006; Goodwin 2010). However, the success of telehealth and telecare is multifaceted, and while technological advances are occurring at an unprecedented level and an evidence base for its effectiveness is growing as a result of the WSD trial (Steventon 2012), it is important to remember that technology, no matter how effective, will not 'do' things by itself. The dissemination and effective use of assistive technology is dependent on an appropriately trained workforce.

According to Goodwin (2010) approximately 1.7 million people benefit from telehealth services in the UK; however, only 5,000 are using them, many of whom received services through the WSD trial. Goodwin (2010) identifies a number of barriers to telehealth implementation, including the implications for health care professionals and organisations of changing their established methods of practice, and suggests more education and research are needed when attempting to implement new technologies. Leonard (2004) states that despite volumes of research pertaining to new technology, research on how best to use it results primarily in frustration, for little has been done to facilitate the adoption of technology in health care. Perednia and Allen (1995) suggest that the ultimate success of telehealth requires that an adopting organisation addresses not only technological, but also managerial challenges, including user technology acceptance, and according to Carneiro (2006) when adopting new technologies organisations should focus on learning, teamwork, knowledge sharing and innovation just as much as the technology itself.

Cantor, Chittamooru and Nobel (2006) warn that as technological advancements continue to develop and provide solutions to caregiving needs, without the education and support of health and social care practitioners they will fail to reach their potential. Organisations need to recognise that assistive technologies may not be that compelling unless health and social care practitioners have mastered the operation of what is available to them and, with such diverse systems and approaches, it is essential that practitioners receive effective education and training when using technology, ensuring appropriate interpretation of data collected (Horwitz et al. 2008).

Although it is recognised by organisations that practitioners have a critical role in the deployment and use of assistive technologies, little attention has been devoted to determining HSCP (Health and Social Care Partnership (Scotland)) training and education (Cantor 2006). Hasman (1998) provides a distinction between training and education within care. He describes training as the immediate knowledge and skills required in the near future and education as long-term knowledge and skills development motivating learning and problem solving. The successful implementation of assistive technologies is dependent on the skills and knowledge of the practitioner, therefore it is important that staff are not only trained to use the technology but also have the educational foundations to understand the theoretical underpinnings, facilitating a link between theory and practice. Skills for Care (2013) published a learning and development framework, resource hub and an app to help ensure that the workforce is capable, confident and skilled in helping people who need care and support make the most of the opportunities that assistive technology can offer them. Similarly, Skills for Health have developed National Occupational Standards for assistive technology (Skills for Health 2014) to describe the skills, knowledge and understanding needed to undertake a particular task or job to a nationally recognised level of competence. They focus on what the person needs to be able to do, as well as what they must know and understand to work effectively.

These initiatives will help develop the current workforce; however, the relevant principles and methods of the use of assistive technology need to be integrated into health and social care undergraduate curriculum ensuring future practitioners are able to understand, accept and utilise technologies to achieve maximal benefit and incorporate them into routine practice (Murphy et al. 2004; Cantor 2005). Unfortunately, there is little research available for descriptions related to curricula and the use of assistive technology, indicating more research needs to be done. Without appropriate training and education programmes there is a danger that a greater gap will emerge between the theoretical and practical application of technology, resulting in abandonment of technology, which will not only have financial implications but also impact on patient and client care.

It is clear that health and social care curriculum development needs to catch up with technological development; however, in the short term other opportunities for training and education are available. Technologies available, but used in other fields, such as simulation, may be translated into assistive technology applications and offer opportunities for training development for health and social care professionals (Conde et al. 2010). Probably the most widely quoted definition of simulation is provided by Gaba (2004) who describes simulation as 'a technique – not a technology – to replace or amplify real experiences with guided experiences that evoke or replicate substantial aspects of the real world in a fully interactive manner'. Simulation aims to provide the learner with opportunities to acquire essential skills in an environment that closely resembles real life. Simulated technologies, including simulated human patients and artificial intelligence applications (second life), offer opportunities for the simulation of real case scenarios in a realistic environment encouraging practitioners to apply their knowledge to practical situations.

Training in the use of assistive technology could include simulation as an active learning strategy, allowing the learners to engage with technology and understand its implementation by combining training with education. Simulation offers many advantages to learners by allowing errors to be made in a safe environment, improving confidence, enhancing decision-making skills, improving psychomotor, technical and teamworking skills and encouraging effective communication (Gaba 2004). Without strategies such as simulation bridging the gap between theory and practice there is a concern that health and social care staff may become reliant upon technologies to inform decision-making, creating complacency with regard to risks and responsibilties (Stanberry 2000). According to Stanberry (2000), the risks to patient privacy and confidentiality and other ethical concerns such as professional accountabilty when using assitive technologies is a barrier to its implementation: 'we have been been so impressed with what we could technically do that we had stopped thinking about how we should ethically be doing it ' (p. 620). Simulation may not provide all the training and education needs for health and social care practitioners but evidence from other health education programmes such as medicine and nursing supports the use of simulation, and thus they have included this experiental teaching method within curricula. Ethical implications can be incorporated into simulated scenarios providing an understanding of the issues and impact on user safety. Simulation in health care is not a new initiative however, advances in simulated technology offer superb learning opportunities and encourage a more interprofessional approach to health and social care education (CMO 2008).

Barr (2001) defines interprofessional education as

> The application of principles of adult learning to interactive, group based learning, which relates collaborative learning to collaborative practice within a coherent rationale which is informed by understanding of interpersonal, group, organisational and inter organisational relations and processes of professionalization'. Assistive technology service innovations are delivered by cross agency partnerships, involving many authorities and practitioners, however, there is little in the way of shared knowledge and expertise.

According to Stanberry (2000), embedding new technologies to support people with both health and social care needs is unlikely to meet its full potential unless the system itself accepts the need to integrate assistive technology into services, and suggests that stakeholders need to consider new ways of working to be successful. Fong, Fong and Li (2011) suggest that a uniform change across all services is of vital importance for a swift switch to making good use of available technology.

The future of digitally enabled reablement services

What does the future look like for digitally enabled reablement services? Homes of the future have been talked about since the 1950s where the vision for home automation was one in which technology was integrated in such a way as to make life easier for the occupants, and this fits well with the concept of reablement. High-tech appliances and gadgets are now not only aimed exclusively at wealthy consumers but already feature in the everyday lives of families. Intelligent home automation linked to digital TV and mobile technology as a means of accessing services and information is becoming more common (Awang and Ward 2011).

Recent developments include intelligent, wireless lighting control systems such as that available from Cybersytems (www.cyberhomesltd. co.uk) which allow management of all of the lights in a home, matching the user's exact requirements and supporting efficient energy use. Integrated heating and remote energy controls linked to mobile phones are now available as a consumer service – for example, Hive by British Gas (www.hivehome.com) and new consumer-focused assisted living services such the AroundMe™ service that uses existing connected home sensor technologies to detect usual daily routines and SMS messaging to inform family and friends that their loved one is 'OK' (Ward et al. 2014). All offer opportunities for people with long-term conditions living at home to have greater control over their environments or to be supported remotely by informal carers or relatives.

Other technologies in social networking and virtual environments offer unprecedented opportunities for social engagement and interaction outside of the home to support people at risk of isolation and loneliness. This is an aspect that was given a lot of attention in previous chapters. Robotics, in terms of exoskeletons to replace lost function and movement, are becoming a reality. Exoskeleton developers working in rehabilitation are leading the way in creating wearable robotic suits that allow people with lower-limb paralysis to walk upright again (Mohammed and Amirat 2012). Smart clothing and internal body sensors to monitor health and well-being are becoming a reality, and in the future who knows how health and social care practice will be changed because of these developments, but at this present time technology offers new choices and opportunities for how people are supported to regain skills and independence within their own homes. Practitioners must equip themselves with the skills and knowledge needed to be able to support service users in that choice.

Summary

> Mainstream and specialist technologies can support and enhance reablement services.

> There is an evidence base for the use of such technologies.

> Technology has the potential to optimise people's independence.

> There are challenges in the acceptability of technologies.

> Adequate staff training in the assessment for, and provision of technologies, is paramount.

Recommended reading

AWANG, D. & WARD, G. (2011) Assistive Technology – A means of empowerment in long term conditions: A guide for nurses and healthcare professionals. In S. Randall and H. Ford (eds). *Long-term conditions: A guide for nurses and healthcare professionals.* Oxford: Blackwell Publishing.

FONG, B., FONG, A. C. M. & LI, C. K. (2011) *Telemedicine technologies: Information technologies in medicine and health.* West Sussex: Wiley.

References

AGE UK (n.d.) *Technology and Older Peoples Evidence Review.* Available at: http://www.ageuk.org.uk/documents/en-gb/for-professionals/computers-and-technology/evidence_review_technology.pdf?dtrk=true (Accessed 15 January 2014).

ASSOCIATION OF DIRECTORS OF ADULT SOCIAL SERVICES (2013) *Social Care funding is getting bleaker.* May. Available at: http://www.adass.org.uk/index.php?option=com_content&id=914&Itemid=489 (Accessed 12 December 2013).

AWANG, D. & WARD, G. (2011) *Assistive Technology – A means of empowerment in long term conditions: A guide for nurses and healthcare professionals.* In S. Randall and H. Ford (eds). *Long-term conditions: A guide for nurses and healthcare professionals.* Oxford: Blackwell Publishing.

BARR, H. (2001) *Inter professional education, today, yesterday and tomorrow.* Learning and teaching support network centre for health sciences and practice from the UK centre for advancement of inter professional education. London.

BURKE, S. (2010) *A better life: Alternative approaches from the perspective of families and carers of older people with high support needs.* Joseph Rowntree Foundation. Available at: https://www.jrf.org.uk/report/better-life-alternative-approaches-perspective-families-and-carers-older-people-high-support (Accessed 12 December 2017).

CANTOR, M. D., CHITTAMOORU, S. & NOBEL, J. (2005) *Training healthcare professionals to use telehealth technology: The missing link.* Available at: http://www.aaai.org/Papers/Symposia/Fall/2005/FS-05-02/FS05-02-004.pdf (Accessed on 13 December 2013).

CARERS UK (2013) *The potential for change. Transforming public awareness of health & care technology.* London: Carers UK.

CARNEIRO, A. (2006) Adopting new technologies. *Handbook of business strategy.* vol. 7, no. 1, 307–312.

CHAU, P. Y. K. & HU, A. J. H. (2002) Investigating healthcare professionals' decisions to accept telemedicine technology: An empirical test of competing theories. *Information & Management,* vol. 39, 279–311.

COCHRANE LIBRARY (2010) *Telemedicine.* Special Collection. Available at: http://www.cochranelibrary.com/app/content/special-collections/article/?doi=10.1002/(ISSN)14651858(CAT)na(VI)SC000013 (Accessed 12 December 2013).

CONDE, J. G., SUVRANU, D., HALL, R. H., JOHANSEN, E., MEGLAN, D. & PENG, G. C. Y. (2010) Telehealth innovations in health education and training. *Telemedicine and eHealth,* vol. 16, 103–106.

DAVIS, F. (1989) User Acceptance of Computer Technology: A comparison of two theoretical models. *Management Science,* vol. 35, 982–1003. Cited in EduTechWiki (2012) *Technology Acceptance.* Available at: http://edutechwiki.unige.ch/en/Technology_acceptance_model (Accessed 5 December 2013).

DH (DEPARTMENT OF HEALTH). (2005) *Building Telecare in England.* Available at: http://webarchive.nationalarchives.gov.uk/+/http://dh.gov.uk/prod_consum_dh/groups/dh_digitalassets/@dh/@en/documents/digitalasset/dh_4115644.pdf (Accessed on 12 December 2013).

DH (DEPARTMENT OF HEALTH). (2006) *Our Health, Our Life, Our Say.* London: HMSO.

DH (DEPARTMENT OF HEALTH). (2009). *150 years of the Annual Report of the Chief Medical Officer: Safer Medical Practice, Machines, Manikins and Polo Mints.* London: HMSO.

DH (DEPARTMENT OF HEALTH). (2011) *Whole System Demonstrator Programme.* Headline Findings, December. Available at: https://www.gov.uk/government/uploads/system/uploads/attachment_data/file/215264/dh_131689.pdf (Accessed 12 December 2013).

DH (DEPARTMENT OF HEALTH). (2014) Care Act 2014. Available at: http://www.legislation.gov.uk/ukpga/2014/23/contents/enacted (Accessed 28 October 2017).

DOUGHTY, K. (2011) SPAs (smartphone applications) – a new form of assistive technology. *Journal of Assistive Technologies,* vol. 5, no. 2, 88–94.

DOUGHTY, K., MONK, A., BAYLISS, C., BROWN, S., DEWSBURY, L., DUNK, B., GALLAGHER, V., GRAFHAM, K., JONES, M., LOWE, C., MCALISTER, L., MCSORLEY, K., MILLS, K., SKIDMORE, C., STEWART, A., TAYLOR B. & WARD, D. (2007) Telecare, telehealth and assistive technologies: Do we know what we are talking about? *Journal of Assistive Technologies,* vol. 1, no. 2, 6–10.

FONG, B., FONG, A. C. M. & LI, C. K. (2011) Telemedicine technologies. *Information technologies in medicine and health.* West Sussex. Wiley.

GABA, D. M. (2004) The future vision of simulation in health care. *Quality and Safety in Health Care,* vol. 12, no. 1, 11–18.

GOODWIN, N. (2010) The state of telehealth and telecare in the UK: Prospects for integrated care. *Journal of Integrated Care,* vol. 18, no. 6, 3–10.

HASMAN, A. (1998) Education and health informatics. *International Journal of Medical Informatics,* vol. 52, no. 1, 209–216.

HORWITZ, C. M., MUELLER, M., WILEY, D., TENTLER, A., BOCKO, M., CHEN, L., LEIBOVICI, A., QUINN, J., SHAR, A. & PENTLAND, A. P. (2008) Is home health technology adequate for proactive self-care? *Methods of Information in Medicine,* vol. 47, no. 1, 58–62.

HSJ (HEALTH SERVICE JOURNAL). (2012) Telehealth: We have the technology, the changing face of health care delivery. *Health Service Journal*, vol. 24, no. 1, 1853–1897. Available at: http://www.hsj.co.uk/Journals/2012/11/28/i/y/j/TELEHEALTHSUPP_121129.pdf (Accessed 5 December 2012).

IPSOS Mediact (2013) Our mobile planet: United Kingdom - Understanding the mobile customer. Available at: http://services.google.com/fh/files/misc/omp-2013-uk-en.pdf (Accessed 4 February 2018).

JANA, R. (2009) How tech for the disabled is going mainstream. *Bloomberg Business Week*, 23 September.

JARROLD, K. & YANDLE, S. (2009) *'A weight off my mind', exploring the impact and potential benefits of telecare for unpaid carers in Scotland.* Glasgow: Carers Scotland.

LEGISLATION.CO.UK. (2000) National Health Service and Community Care Act 1990. Reprint. Available at: https://www.legislation.gov.uk/ukpga/1990/19/pdfs/ukpga_19900019_en.pdf (Accessed 2 December 2017).

LEONARD, K. J. (2004) Critical success factors relating to healthcare's adoption of new technology: A guideline to increasing the likelihood of successful implementation. *Electronic Healthcare*, vol. 2, 74–80.

LINDSAY, S. (2013) *The Ambient Kitchen 2.0: Situated sensing for independent living with cognitive impairment.* Available at: http://stadium.open.ac.uk/webcast-ou/documents/20130205_LINDSAY_-_The_Ambient_Kitchen_2.pdf (Accessed 5 December 2012).

MEDICAL DEVICES AGENCY. (1995) *Environmental control systems. An evaluation.* Disability Equipment Assessment No. A414. Norwich: HMSO.

MILNE, A. & SEABROOKE, V. (2004) *Culture and care in dementia – A study of the Asian community in North West Kent.* Alzheimers and Dementia support services.

MOHAMMED, S. & AMIRAT, Y. H. (2012) Lower-limb movement assistance through wearable robots: State of the art and challenges. *Advanced Robotics*, vol. 26, no. 1/2, 1–22.

MPT (MATCHING PERSON AND TECHNOLOGY) (2013) *Matching Person and Technology (MPT)* Assessment Process. Available at: http://www.matchingpersonandtechnology.com/mptdesc.html (Accessed 5 December 2012).

MURPHY, J., STRAMER, K., CLAMP, S., GRUBB, P., GOSLAND, J. & DAVIS, S. (2004) Health informatics education for clinicians and managers – What's holding up the progress? *International Journal of Medical Informatics*, vol. 73, no. 2, 205–213.

THE NATIONAL ARCHIVES (2010) *Secretary of State for Health's speech to the 5th International Carers Conference – 'The principles of social care reform'.* DH. Available at: http://webarchive.nationalarchives.gov.uk/+/www.dh.gov.uk/en/MediaCentre/Speeches/DH_117331 (Accessed 23 November 2015).

NURSING AND MIDWIFERY COUNCIL. (2007) *Simulation and Practice Learning Project: Outcome of a pilot study to the test principles for auditing simulated practice learning environments in the pre-registration nursing programme.* London: Nursing and Midwifery Council.

OLIVER, P., MONK, A., XU, G. & HOEY, J. (n.d.) *Ambient Kitchen: Designing situated services using a high fidelity prototyping environment.* Available at: http://di.ncl.ac.uk/publicweb/publications/Olivier09ABRA.pdf (Accessed 5 December 2012).

OPM & NEIEP (NORTH EAST IMPROVEMENT AND EFFICIENCY PARTNER-SHIP). (2010) *Reablement: guide for frontline staff.* Available at: https://www.opm.co.uk/wp-content/uploads/2014/01/NEIEP-reablement-guide.pdf (Accessed 12 December 2013).

PEREDNIA, D. A. & ALLEN, A. (1995) Telemedicine technology and clinical applications. *Journal of the American Medical Association*, vol. 273, no. 6, 483–488.

ROYAL COLLEGE OF NURSING (2013) *Telehealth and telecare.* Available at: https://www2.rcn.org.uk/development/practice/e-health/telehealth_and_tele care (Accessed 12 December 2013).

ROYAL COMMISSION ON LONG TERM CARE (1999) *With respect to old age: Research Volume 2.* London: The Stationery Office. http://webarchive.nationalarchives.gov.uk/20131205101144/http://www.archive.official-documents.co.uk/document/cm41/4192/4192.htm (Accessed 17 December 2013).

SCIE (SOCIAL CARE INSTITUTE FOR EXCELLENCE). (2010) *At a glance 24: Ethical issues for the use of telecare.* Available at: http://www.scie.org.uk/publications/ataglance/ataglance24.asp (Accessed 5 May 2012).

SCIE (SOCIAL CARE INSTITUTE FOR EXCELLENCE). (2013) *Fair Access to Care.* Available at: http://www.scie.org.uk/publications/guides/guide33/files/guide33.pdf (Accessed 5 May 2012).

SKILLS FOR CARE (2013) *Assisted Living Technologies, Knowledge and Skills Framework.* Available at: http://www.skillsforcare.org.uk/Skills/Assisted-Living-Technologies/Assisted-living-technology.aspx (Accessed 5 December 2012).

SKILLS FOR HEALTH (2014) *NOS Assistive Technologies.* Available at: http://www.skillsforhealth.org.uk/about-us/competences%10national-occupational-standards/national-occupational-standards-for-assistive-technologies/ (Accessed 21 January 2014).

SMALLMAN, G. (2012) The benefit of apps in healthcare. *Guardian Professional*, 21 August. Available at: https://www.theguardian.com/healthcare-network/2012/aug/21/apps-healthcare-tablets-mobile-smartphones. (Accessed 15 January 2018).

STANBERRY, B. (2000) Telemedicine: Barriers and opportunities in the 21st century. *Journal of Internal Medicine*, vol. 247, no. 6, 615–628.

STEVENTON, A., BARDSLEY, M., BILLINGS, J., DIXON, J., DOLL, H., BENYON, M., HIRANI, S., CARTRIGHT, M., RIXON, L., KNAPP, M., HENDERSON, C., ROGERS, A., FITZPATRICK, R., HENDY, J. & NEWMAN, S. (2012) Effect of telehealth on use of secondary care and mortality: Findings from the Whole System Demonstrator cluster randomised trial. *British Medical Journal*, 344: e3874.

STEVENTON, A., BARDSLEY, M., BILLINGS, J., DIXON, J., DOLL, H., BENYON, M., HIRANI, S., CARTRIGHT, M., RIXON, L., KNAPP, M., HENDERSON, C., ROGERS, A., HENDY, J., FITZPATRICK, R. & NEWMAN, S. (2013) Effect of telecare on use of health and social care services: Findings from the Whole Systems Demonstrator cluster randomised trial. *Age and Ageing*. vol. 42, no. 4, 501–508.

TECHNOLOGY STRATEGY BOARD. (2011) *DALLAS Delivering assisted living lifestyle at scale.* Available at: https://connect.innovateuk.org/documents/3217986/3747519/DALLAS+Competition+Paper.pdf/e35f29a5-7dd4-4945-9bc9-7e5f64abb93f (Accessed December 2014).

VENKATESH, V., MORRIS, M. G., DAVIS, F. D. & DAVIS, G. B. (2003) 'User acceptance of information technology': Toward a unified view. *MIS Quarterly*, vol. 27, no. 3, 425–478. Available at: https://nwresearch.wikispaces.com/file/view/Venkatesh+User+Acceptance+of+Information+Technology+2003.pdf (Accessed 15 January 2018).

WARD, G., HOLLIDAY, N., AWANG, D. & HARSON, D. (2014) Technology and informal care networks: Creative approaches to user led service design for the Warm Neighbourhoods® AroundMe™ service. *Interdisciplinary Studies Journal*, vol. 3, no. 4, 24–31.

WHERTON, J. P. & MONK, A. F. (2008) Technological opportunities for supporting people with dementia who are living at home. *International Journal of Human-Computer Studies*, vol. 66, no. 8, 571–586.

YI, M. Y., JACKSON, J. D., PARK, J. S. & PROBST, J. C. (2006) Understanding information technology acceptance by individual professionals: Towards an integrative view. *Information & Management*, vol. 43, no. 3, 350–363.

YORK HEALTH ECONOMICS CONSORTIUM AT YORK UNIVERSITY & THE SCOTTISH GOVERNMENT (2009) *Evaluation of the Telecare Development Programme* – Final Report. Edinburgh: Scottish Government.

Conclusion

V. Ebrahimi and H. M. Chapman

Any activity involving people is complex. The way we think, feel, behave and interact with each other is demonstrated in the activities we carry out day to day. This can only be partially understood by other people. Our lives are also affected by our interactions with the environment in which we live and the people with whom we share it, as well as the demands and opportunities of wider society. Whether we need support, are involved in supporting others or are interdependent, there will be many influences on the person and the way he/she/we engage with others. As a consequence, there can never be only one way of caring for someone. This is why the principles of reablement, working with a person and their family to help them take control of their lives and achieve their full potential, are so important in meeting the challenges inherent in our changing society. It is also important in our understanding of how certain occupations have meaning to one person but not to another.

Long-term care within institutions is neither desirable nor cost-effective on a large scale, but we cannot expect people to recover from acute episodes of illness or overcome disability to regain autonomy without a bridging service – life is not that simple. Nonetheless, for a long time, services have been trying to manage people's care needs as if it were – simply modifying home care services and discharge processes. This is somewhat understandable given the need to cope with an increasing tide of demand and higher expectations of health and social care support. Placing people in 'social contexts' such as day centres and then reporting that a need for interaction has been met is a false dichotomy in some, if not most, instances. The increasing demand for hospital beds and social care, in a society where independence from the state is valued, has led to the view that we have the problem of an ageing population. This is despite the evidence that older people contribute greatly to the economic and social wealth of our respective countries. Irrespective of this, age and infirmity should not lessen someone's value to us and society at large. Reablement helps people to realise not only their functional potential, but also their human potential. Valuing of the individual and their perspective must be central to the philosophy and practice of reablement.

Interestingly, this latter point on individuality gave rise to some tension among us editors in relation to the use of the term 'service users'. Much debate about an alternative arose, simply because our aim throughout has been to draw on and respect the principles of person-centredness. There is an implicit notion that a person who 'uses' services may be a drain on us, society and our resources – whereas the argument in Chapter 2 is that older people are our economy. We conceded, however, that we must honour the term, not just for ease of reading and understanding, but because there may be a risk of taking too strong a political stance. At times, we were drawn to the terms 'people', 'person' and 'individual' as reference. The term service user, however, seems accepted in the social care context. Perhaps we need to ask older people what suits them best. Then again, this may simply be professional insecurity at play and the name may be of no consequence whatsoever.

Another contention was the use of independence and, more often than not, readers see the term 'autonomy' used throughout. Once more, this is because the alternative term, independence/independent, is bandied about in a practice context – often to the extent of forgetting that independence has different meanings to different people. Stating that someone has autonomy denotes a better sense of control over that person's individual dislikes and likes – whether they are happy with the outcome. Chapter 4 included a discussion as to how traditional approaches to care can create a culture of dependency. Whether someone is independent or not is a decision often made by the practitioner or support worker. It was thus important to have some debate on what we understand the term independence to mean and how this differs to autonomy. This was discussed in quite some depth in both Chapters 4 and 7. Significantly, high-tech advances such as assistive devices and smart technologies were explored in Chapter 8. How these might be used in reablement services alongside the supporting evidence was also examined. The concerns that assistive devices might increase isolation, alongside positive aspects, such as how technologies can be empowering, were also illustrated.

An important addition that must be included here is our reference throughout the book to unpaid carers and definitions that were outlined in Chapter 1. We do not mean that by calling carers 'informal' that their contribution is not of value. This is by no means meant to diminish their role or status – far from it. It was considered to allow a better contrast between the more formal paid carer, the carer who has no intimate connection and is paid to 'care for'. We also had to make a distinction between formal carers and reablement support workers; both are paid, yet they have a markedly different approach in their practice and associated role.

This understanding of human complexity, along with a commitment to engaging people in meaningful activity, means that anyone who works in reablement needs a wide range of skills and knowledge to perform and evaluate their role. This book examined the role of the support worker in Chapter 5. They are the lynchpin in the reablement process, ensuring there is a fit between the needs of the individual and the resources of family, friends, community and health and social care professionals. However, they can also help individuals and their social networks to recognise their value. An older person, or a person with a disability or long-term condition, may have time to think about other people and offer them time for conversation and companionship. They may have interesting stories or viewpoints on life, or skills or knowledge that they can share. They have their own personalities, life goals and experiences. The support worker can uncover these, finding opportunities for purposeful activities that bring added meaning to them, the people around them and society at large. Society, in its largest sense, does not always value the achievement of a person, but that person gains reward from achievement of their goals and from good relationships with those around them. This applies to both service users and support workers – by valuing the people we work with, we value ourselves; and by achieving our goals through helping others to achieve theirs, we gain a sense of satisfaction from a good job well done.

The historical context of reablement and how this affects models of service provision today was considered in Chapter 3. Other professionals, people and their families may not be familiar with the concept of reablement, but understanding its service and philosophical origins and the different modes of service delivery will give reablement workers confidence in explaining their role within the service to colleagues and the people that use them. In order to justify and evaluate the effectiveness of reablement, it is important to understand the meaning and implications of research studies and be able to take part in any audits or evaluations of reablement services. As research is still limited in reablement, it has not been discussed here in much depth. It is anticipated, however, that another text in the near future will outline the core principles of research, its methodology and the national and international studies that bring added value to the practice domain.

Chapter 6 identified the importance of reablement in helping people and their informal carers to manage long-term conditions. It discussed examples of possible scenarios and practical ways in which reablement workers can make a difference to people's ability to manage their lives in a more autonomous manner. Previous care experiences, however, may be a barrier to the independence of a person, requiring the reablement service, with its philosophy of person-centred approaches, to support activity and independence within an informal care network. This was supported by an examination of the reasons why older people and those with disabilities may feel devalued, and how individual interactions with other people have the potential to enhance their self-esteem, with a consequent effect on both their quality of life and physical well-being. Chapter 7 also discussed how, under the influence of culturally held negative views, people may not value older or disabled people, with serious negative effects on how the person views themselves and ultimately their physical and mental well-being. These views were challenged and the reader was given the opportunity to reflect on their own thoughts, feelings and behaviours related to stigmatising features, both in themselves and in others.

It is essential for its success for all involved to understand that reablement is not merely a renamed service, with slightly more specialised practitioners who can call on more resources. This is a process that involves, at its core, the relationship between two people. It is the change in the nature of that relationship that underpins the whole process of reablement. We all agree essentially, and call for a mind shift, not only in health and social care but by society at large, to alter the way in which we perceive our older community-dwelling adults. Of course, this has to start somewhere and where better than in the way in which formal care is provided.

So ... can reablement achieve this? Will we work towards co-production, providing opportunities for engagement in meaningful activities of choice, facilitating people towards autonomy and well-being? We leave you here to contemplate these questions, but not before this eloquent reminder from Ellen Langer. We could not help but add our own addition to it because it sums up so well the idea of what reablement means to us:

> *'Ageing means change, but change does not mean decay'* (Langer 2009, p. 256)
>
> ... *it is just growth in a new direction.*

Reference

LANGER, E. (2009) *Counter-clockwise: Mindful health and the power of possibility.* London: Hodder & Stoughton.

Glosssary

Active listening A conscious effort to listen not only to the content of what people are saying, but also the meaning it has for them. The active listener develops their understanding of what someone is saying and then reflects it back to them, checking that they understand what it means to that. person. Active listening demonstrates engagement with the person and is fundamental to a therapeutic relationship with them.

Activity A component of occupation – something that needs to be undertaken in order to achieve occupational goals. Meaningful activities are fundamental to an enhanced quality of live. Activity and occupation are closely related to health and well-being.

Activity analysis Occurs when a task is broken down into various components and then analysed in terms of the abilities required to carry out a task.

Activity theory of ageing Suggests the maintenance of earlier active patterns of life is associated with successful retirement and that activity helps physical and psychological well-being.

Acute conditions Conditions that generally develop quickly, are short term, cause severe symptoms and are potentially life-threatening.

Advocacy Formal advocacy is provided by an advocate (usually independent) who represents the person in ensuring that health and social care decisions and care are made according to their wishes or, if they cannot be known, in their best interests. This includes helping them to gain access to information and services, being involved in discussions about care, exploring choices, promoting their rights and speaking out on important issues. Advocacy is particularly important to people who are vulnerable and may need safeguarding, such as older people, people with mental health problems, people with learning disabilities and people who are physically frail.

Ageing in place A term used to describe a person living in the residence of their choice, for as long as they are able, as they age. This includes being able to have any services (or other support) they might need over time as their needs change (Ageinplace.com 2015).

Ageism A form of discrimination that is based on a person's age. Age is one of the protected characteristics of The Equality Act (2010), along with disability, gender reassignment, marriage and civil partnership, race, religion or belief, sex, sexual orientation, meaning that it is illegal to discriminate against people on these grounds, either directly (treat someone less favourably) or indirectly (where an organisation's practices, policies or procedures result in disadvantaging an older person).

Agorophobia An intense real fear in an individual when going out into open spaces. This can be experienced even when there are no people around.

Assistive technology A device or system that enables someone to be independent in certain activities or to be safer through the use of technology.

Autonomic nervous system The part of the nervous system that regulates the function of internal organs, and is mostly under unconscious (hence autonomic) control. It is regulated by the hypothalamus, and consists of the sympathetic and the parasympathetic nervous systems, controlling heart rate, digestion, respiratory rate, pupillary response, urination and sexual arousal. It is responsible for the 'fight or flight' and the 'rest and digest' responses.

Autonomy The condition of being free or independent, with the right to make one's own decisions. In health and social care, autonomy of the person is a right that should be upheld by practitioners. In situations where people do not have the mental capacity (see capacity below) to make a choice or decision on a particular issue at a particular time, all appropriate measures must be taken to ensure that any decisions made and care given are in the person's best interests and accord with their wishes.

Backward chaining The carrying out of an activity starting with the last part, to gain immediate reward for effort.

Bipolar Disorder A term used in psychiatry for a condition where a person can have extreme highs or euphoria (manic stage) or lows (depressive stage) which interfere with daily life. Sometimes at risk to self and on occasion others.

Blurring Used often to define something that does not have a definitive boundary. In health and social care this might be the blurring of roles such as the ability for nurses, physiotherapists and occupational therapists to prescribe medication.

Capability Having ability or having the potential to develop a characteristic. In the context of reablement: Separated into two domains - 'functionings' and 'capabilities'. Functionings refers to doing or ways of being wheras capabilities are demonstrable when an individual has genuine opportunities to achieve these functions. See Entwistle & Watt (2013) Treating patients as persons: A capabilities approach to support delivery of person-centred care. Available from: https://www.ncbi.nlm.nih.gov/pmc/articles/PMC3746461/ (Accessed 4 February 2018).

Capacity [and consent] The ability of someone to do something or understand what they are doing. Consent results in a decision based on this understanding.

Cardiovascular accident (CVA) Damage caused by either a clot in the blood supply to the brain or, less commonly, by a bleed out of the blood vessel into the brain. In either case, brain cells (neurones) die due to a lack of oxygen.

Care scheme Known also as a 'package of care' which includes agreed support by paid carers who assist with personal care or domestic tasks. Often but not always organised by a social worker/social care assessor or as part of a personal budget.

Chunking A technique where an activity is broken down into manageable amounts.

Clinical commissioning group These consist of GP managers who are responsible for deciding what proportion of received funds will be allocated to which services. These allocations comprise hospital and community

NHS services in local areas but more specifically to rehabilitative care and community health.

Clinical supervision A discussion of practice issues and critical incidents with a qualified team leader, in the form of a supported reflection on their educational development, managerial support and psychological needs.

Clinical reasoning skills The use of existing knowledge, skills and prior experience of situations which are brought to the forefront during interactions with a person or other interdisciplinary members involved in their care.

Clonus Rapid involuntary stiffening and loosening of muscles, as seen sometimes with spasticity.

Co-production A meeting of minds coming together to find a shared solution. In practice, it involves people who use services being consulted, included and working together from the start to the end of any project that affects them.

Cognitive Abilities related to thinking and processing thought, such as memory, attention, understanding, learning.

Cognitive behavioural therapy Therapists will sometimes use this approach to alter the way a person thinks about a situation to ultimately change the behaviours which interfere with daily life.

Cognitive reframing The assessment of negative thoughts to see if they are accurate, or if there is another, more balanced, perspective.

Compensation and/or compensatory methods in reablement Compensation is a learned behaviour to alleviate pain or discomfort. For example, instead of using the left hand (stroke) the right is consistently used. To undo this, a compensatory method in reablement might involve encouragement to use the right hand more; for instance, to pick up items with it when cooking.

Concept An idea, notion or model for thinking about something.

Concordance Describes a partnership approach between a person and service provider leading to a mutual understanding and shared goals.

Conditional positive regard Valuing the person only when their behaviour conforms to expectations. This can result in incongruence.

Congruence/authenticity A state where a person's view of themselves as they are (self-image) and the way they would like to be (ideal self) are very similar, so the person feels happy with who they are. Congruence or authenticity is a state of self-awareness and openness in which the person presents a genuine version of themselves to others, resulting in trustworthiness.

Continuing professional development All professions are required through their code of conduct to keep up to date with changing and/or current practice. Often in the form of a journal club, individual reflection and sometimes study, attendance at internal or external training, or conferences.

Debate A process during discussions on which course of action or system is best by considering different aspects and views on the matter.

Depersonalising The process of undermining a person's individual identity by not valuing them and not listening or responding to their views.

Dichotomy In a discussion (discourse) about something it means that there are contradictions or that there is an irreconcilable or incompatible difference.

Discreditable A trait that is perceived as harmful to one's reputation or blameworthy. See stigma.

Disengagement theory People gradually withdraw from more powerful roles in society, focusing more on close family on friends, to prevent disruption to society when they die, and to reduce the stress and strain of leading a fuller life.

Dressing stick A stick with a hook on the end to help with picking up and putting on clothes – usually skirts, trousers, dresses.

Dysphagia Difficulty in swallowing.

Empathy Understanding the world from the other person's view in order to relate to their emotional feelings and needs.

Enabling To facilitate someone in, for example, achieving their occupational goals.

Energy conservation Ensuring through technical instruction that the person is aware of and has sufficient energy to carry out tasks autonomously.

Ethos A philosophy or a belief.

Flood detectors Detectors which have sensors that trigger an audible alarm and can link to a system where a carer is alerted by telephone if a flood occurs.

Flow (Csiksentmihalyi, 1990) A state when all sense of time is lost and we lose our sense of self. The mind or body is stretched to its limits in a determined effort to accomplish a task that is difficult and worthwhile.

Formal care Care that is provided by paid support staff from either an external agency (business) or a voluntary, local authority or NHS organisation.

Generic The opposite of specific. An example might be a generic support worker who has an understanding of nursing, physiotherapy and occupational therapy. The worker would draw on these different skills in their role.

Gerotranscendence When the older person makes choices that suit their needs and desires in later life. Often has a spiritual dimension.

Haemorrhagic stroke Bleeding out of a blood vessel in the brain causing a disruption to the blood supply to the brain cells, leading to brain damage.

Helping hand A grab stick which is operated through the use of a trigger in the handle, usually spring loaded.

Hemianopia Visual perception limited to one side of the visual field, usually caused by a cerebral vascular accident (CVA).

Holistic/holistic care Involves taking into account the needs and goals of the whole person, rather than seeing someone in terms of their health and social care needs alone.

Humanistic approach An approach in psychology where the subject of interest is the person as a whole from their own perspective. For example, the expert in what a person needs is the person themselves.

Incongruence Feelings of low self-worth due to experiencing conditional positive regard, leading to a disconnect between one's true inner self and the outer self, resulting in acting a role in order to make oneself likeable to others.

Infantilism Words or actions which are inappropriately expressed and that do not match the age of the person. 'Aww she is just so nice and cuddly' (referring to an 80-year-old woman).

Informal care Unpaid care that is provided by a partner, husband or wife, wider family friend or neighbour. The informal carer may be eligible for a carer's allowance payment (state benefit). The term used here is not to denigrate their role but to differentiate between them and paid carers, – here termed formal care.

Intermediate care An umbrella term for a number of different services which are all based in the community. These include hospital at home; intermediate care units and reablement.

Intervention Any type of face to face contact with a person, be it for assessment, activity enabling, equipment or adaptation provision or review.

Institutionalisation A situation whereby a person who lives with others becomes negatively affected by those in control (often formal carers and professionals) to their detriment. This can have an impact on activities, expression of individuality, sociability, mood and behaviour amongst many other areas.

Kyphosis Curvature of the spine, marked by an abnormally rounded upper back. This particularly affects respiratory function and mobility.

Learned helplessness The effect of previous experiences of failure leading to a belief that future efforts are hopeless and therefore not worth attempting.

Meta-analysis Statistical approach to combining the data from a number of studies to increase the strength of the findings.

Metaphorical Not a literal sense but rather a figure of speech.

Mindfulness Paying attention to what is happening within and around us.

Mortality The state of being mortal and the inevitability of death.

Neuropsychological processing The way in which the brain processes thoughts, feelings and perceptions and responds to them.

Occupation There are about four sub-sets of this: daily activity, work, leisure and play.

Outcomes-based approach Assessing interventions by their effectiveness rather than by the time they take.

Paradigm [shift] One way of thinking about a concept. When it shifts we change our way of thinking about something to another.

Perception A specific psychological term which is the conscious awareness of internal and external stimuli. Processing and interpreting sensory stimuli.

Personal assistant An individual who is assigned to another in the context of care.

Personal budget Personalised funds to enable an individual to choose what assistance they would like.

Person-centred (chapter 6) Working with people to identify their needs, motivations and abilities, ensuring that they are able to make fully-informed choices and have control over the process.

Person-centred (Carl Rogers, chapter 8) This approach is based on the view that the person knows their own problems and needs better than anyone else, so the helper must provide conditions of growth to allow them to identify these. Conditions of growth involve empathising with the person's perspective, providing them with unconditional positive regard and being authentic (or congruent), so that they feel secure and able to express themselves. See congruence.

Person-Centred Planning A care plan which is written from the perspective of the person.

Phenomenon An occurrence or observable experience.

Philosophy A way of understanding the world or a belief system.

Pill dispensers An automated system which contains the required medication and is set to provide an alarm at times when the medication is required.

Policy A system of principles that guide decision-making to ensure standardised approaches.

Positioning A term used in kinesiology which refers to the correct posture or stance prior to engaging in movement, walking and any activity.

Post-modern Life cannot be understood as one truth but as a set of subjective truths depending on the presence and perspective of an observer. Status and power are not necessarily seen as legitimate or dependent on having the best attributes.

Primary agents (chapter 1) A fundamental aspect that enables something else to occur. For example, activities are primary agents in all human beings that facilitate exploration and learning.

Pseudonym A different name to the birth name of an individual. Often used to anonymise and protect confidentiality.

Quality of life General well-being of an individual in relation to their daily life.

Radical [reform] When a particular position leads to different thinking and moves away from what is traditional. Something that is progressive or innovative. When radical is associated with reform the intention is to vocalise this through political means or as a social group.

Rapid response Professionals who are often based in A&E or within a community practice team whose aim is to help avoid unnecessary hospital admission. Teams often comprise of an occupational therapist, physiotherapist and nurse or a combination.

Rapport This is based on a two way relationship that needs to develop, often but not always slowly, enabling some kind of mutual understanding of each other's perspective. This occurs during the interactions between professional/support worker and the recipient of an intervention.

Reablement A service which enables a person to carry out a number of different activities despite an impairment, disability or long-term condition. It is also aimed at prevention most commonly with hospital admission. Another objective in reablement may be to reduce or withdraw formal care.

Reablement support worker/s Anyone working in a reablement capacity including interdisciplinary professionals and support staff.

Rehabilitation A method to enable a person to maintain, regain or compensate for disability or difficulties in mobility. This might be resultant from a condition, trauma (hip fracture) or impairment (vision) or long-term or short-term disability.

Resilience The psychological ability to adapt to stress and adverse events.

Restorative/restorative approach Term used internationally to describe reablement but with a difference to the UK usually in length of time and type of enablement interventions.

Secondary healthcare Associated with hospital services, consultants and medical specialism. This is the opposite to primary care (term still in use) which involves services in the community such as GP surgeries, community rehabilitation, reablement and district nursing and physiotherapy.

Self-actualisation/personal growth The process of leading a life in which the person feels happy within themselves but looks forward to the next challenge or opportunity for self-development.

Self-concept The belief we have of ourselves as being a certain sort of person with particular traits, attributes and characteristics.

Self-determination Having control of your situation or self; autonomous.

Self-efficacy The belief that we have control over events in the world (that might include our behaviour).

Sensory Sensation such as touch, smell, hearing, sight, taste.

Service user Individuals who use services whether reablement or otherwise. This is not a preferred term in the book as it is not person-centred however it is commonly used within health and social care services making it easier to distinguish in subsequent discussions.

Social construct A perception of an individual, group or idea that is constructed culturally through social interactions or institutions or processes.

Social discourse Communication that has a social purpose or aspect; particularly important when considering our own feelings towards groups of people within society and whether or not our views are affected by peer groups, the media or influential people.

Social model A framework for understanding concepts such as disability as social constructs rather than personal attributes.

Sock aid An item specifically designed to assist someone to put on their socks without the need to bend.

Spasticity Difficulty in controlling muscles, making them tight or stiff. Reflex movements may be excessively strong or last much longer than usual.

Spike board A board where items to be chopped are held in place by spikes meaning they can be chopped using only one hand.

Spreader board A board with raised edges at the corners which prevent bread from slipping when being buttered.

Stigma A discreditable trait (in some cultural perspectives) that sets a person apart and is often seen as a negative quality by others. Even if people do not actively discriminate against the stigmatised person, that person may behave differently or try to hide their stigmatising trait in order to avoid labelling and potential discrimination.

Subarachnoid haemorrhage A bleed on the surface of the brain causing pressure that if not released leads to brain damage or death.

Successful ageing A position which places importance on life expectancy alongside an absence of deterioration in physical, mental and cognitive ability (Biomedical position). On a different level Psychosocial positions place more emphasis on life satisfaction, social participation and functioning. Yet these positions may not be the same for the lay or older person who may view this as having a sense of purpose; financial security; learning new things; accomplishments; physical appearance; productivity; contribution to life; sense of humour and spirituality.

Supported discharge Known sometimes as 'discharge package' or 'package of care'. The complete support network for a person once they leave hospital or an intermediate care setting. This might include formal and informal care, reablement and other services (such as district nursing), environmental adaptations (rails on walls or ramp at door) and assistive technology.

Support worker Refers to support workers whereas 'reablement workers' (see above) encompasses any member, including those that have been trained by interdisciplinary professionals.

Symbolic interactionism The theory that people derive meaning from social interactions which influences their behaviour towards them. For example, if epilepsy is viewed as a divine judgement, then the person with the condition may be stigmatised and then treated less favourably than others.

Task The component part of an activity. For example, when dressing, one task might be to choose a jumper to match a skirt.

Telehealth Specific technologies that can monitor health at distance. For example, taking blood pressure readings remotely perhaps via a person's television.

Therapeutic relationship Where the relationship between the person and the professional influences the effectiveness of the intervention.

Unconditional positive regard Valuing the person as an end in themselves, regardless of their status or personal characteristics.

Values Something particular that an individual ascribes importance to or worth.

Voluntary movement Initiated movement rather than an involuntary one, which is an automatic uncontrollable movement response (see clonus and spasticity).

Index

In this index *f* represents figure, *t* represents table, and *g* represents glossary

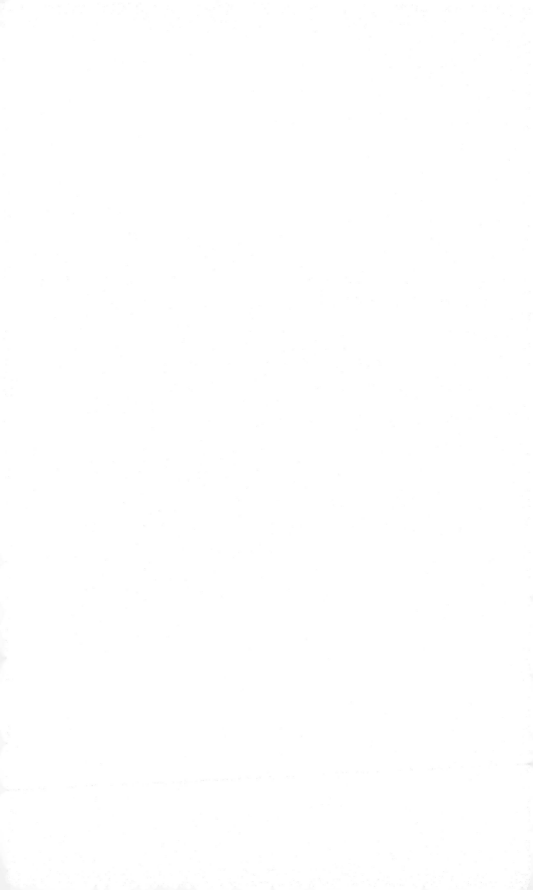

Printed by Printforce, the Netherlands